BEHAVIORAL ACTIVATION
FOR DEPRESSION

BEHAVIORAL ACTIVATION FOR DEPRESSION
A Clinician's Guide

CHRISTOPHER R. MARTELL
SONA DIMIDJIAN
RUTH HERMAN-DUNN

Foreword by Peter M. Lewinsohn

THE GUILFORD PRESS
New York   London

© 2010 The Guilford Press
A Division of Guilford Publications, Inc.
72 Spring Street, New York, NY 10012
www.guilford.com

Printed in the United States of America

This book is printed on acid-free paper.

Last digit is print number: 9 8 7 6 5 4 3

Library of Congress Cataloging-in-Publication Data

Martell, Christopher R.
  Behavioral activation for depression : a clinician's guide / Christopher R. Martell,
Sona Dimidjian, and Ruth Herman-Dunn.
     p. ; cm.
  Includes bibliographical references and index.
  ISBN 978-1-60623-515-7 (hardcover : alk. paper)
  ISBN 978-1-4625-1017-7 (paperback : alk. paper)
  1. Depression, Mental—Treatment. 2. Behavior therapy. I. Dimidjian, Sona. II.
Herman-Dunn, Ruth. III. Title.
  [DNLM: 1. Depressive Disorder—therapy. 2. Cognitive Therapy—methods.
WM 171 M376b 2010]
  RC537.M3737 2010
  616.85′27—dc22
                                            2009040847

*This book is dedicated to the late Neil S. Jacobson,
our friend, colleague, and behavioral activation mentor.*

We are forever indebted to his initial vision for this work.

*Neil's memory influences us in all our research,
writing, and clinical work.*

About the Authors

Christopher R. Martell, PhD, ABPP, is Clinical Associate Professor in the Department of Psychiatry and Behavioral Sciences and in the Department of Psychology at the University of Washington in Seattle, where he also has a private practice. He is board certified in both clinical psychology and behavioral psychology through the American Board of Professional Psychology and is a founding fellow of the Academy of Cognitive Therapy. The coauthor of four books, Dr. Martell has published widely on behavioral treatments for depression and other areas of application of cognitive-behavioral therapy, including cognitive-behavioral therapy with lesbian, gay, and bisexual clients. He is an international workshop leader and lecturer, and was the recipient of the Washington State Psychological Association's Distinguished Psychologist Award in 2004.

Sona Dimidjian, PhD, is Assistant Professor of Psychology at the University of Colorado at Boulder. Her research addresses the treatment and prevention of depression, including a particular focus on the mental health of women during pregnancy and postpartum. Dr. Dimidjian is a leading expert in cognitive and behavioral approaches to treating and preventing depression. She is one of a core group of experts in behavioral activation (BA) treatment for depression and has published widely in this area. Dr. Dimidjian is also an expert in the clinical application of contemplative practices, such as mindfulness meditation, and is an international workshop leader and lecturer.

Ruth Herman-Dunn, PhD, is in private practice in Seattle and supervises graduate students in her position as Clinical Instructor in the Department of Psychology at the University of Washington. She has been a research therapist on several large randomized clinical trials for behavioral treatments, including BA and dialectical behavior therapy, and has led workshops on these treatments throughout the United States and Canada. Dr. Herman-Dunn provides consultation on treatment dissemination studies and collaborates with a core group of BA experts on research, training, and treatment development.

Acknowledgments

There are a number of people who have generously given time and attention to this project to whom we wish to extend our gratitude.

The University of Washington Treatments for Depression Study, in Seattle, was the birthplace of our conceptualization of behavioral activation (BA), and the people involved in that study have been instrumental in guiding our thinking over the past decade. We thank the study's participants and all the clients with whom we have worked since then whose dedication and efforts have inspired and shaped our work. We are grateful to the investigators on the BA study, our dear friends and colleagues Robert J. Kohlenberg, PhD, Steven D. Hollon, PhD, Keith S. Dobson, PhD, Karen B. Schmaling, PhD, Michael E. Addis, PhD, and David L. Dunner, MD. Robert Gallop, PhD, is a statistical genius and an invaluable collaborator as well. Finally, Marsha M. Linehan, PhD, has been an inspiration and guide in many ways. Whether consulting on specific clients or talking about behavior therapy over dinner at her home, she offered keen insights into theory and technique, graciously challenged us to refine our thinking, and shared her enthusiasm for the ongoing importance of this work.

Many conversations over the years with colleagues and friends have also sharpened our thinking and understanding. In particular, Virginia Rutter, PhD, has been an ongoing source of support, friendship, and wisdom. Chris Dunn, PhD, David Markley, PhD, Linda Dimeff, PhD, Sarah Landes, PhD, and Sandra Coffman, PhD, engaged us in stimulating discussions about theory and technique and helped to shape the book without necessarily knowing at the time the valuable contribution they were making. Eric Woodcock, BS, had the original idea for the acronym ACTIVATE and has been a tremendous help and coordinator on several BA-related projects.

Clinicians and researchers Tina Pittman-Wagers, PsyD, Samuel Hubley, BA, and Roselinde Kaiser, MA, polished our final draft and deserve our warmest thanks. JoAnne Dahl, PhD, and Anna Suessbrick, PhD, outstanding scholars and clinicians, gave feedback that allowed us to complete this project with confidence.

We also wish to recognize the important contributions of several individuals at The Guilford Press, including Jim Nageotte, Senior Editor; Jane Keislar, Assistant Editor; Kelly K. Waering, Jr., copy editor; and Louise Farkas, Senior Production Editor. Although they remain anonymous, the reviewers who read our first proposal and initial draft and critically evaluated the project also deserve to be acknowledged for their contributions.

Christopher R. Martell acknowledges Mark E. Williams for being a wonderfully supportive, centering, and caring partner. With his superior writing skills, Mark graciously read and commented on many portions of the text and offered brilliant editorial advice. He also thanks his sisters, Catherine Borkman and Anita Bourgault, and brother, Paul Martell, for support and patience throughout the development of this book.

Sona Dimidjian acknowledges with gratitude Chuck Langdon for being a remarkable partner in life, love, work, and parenting; his support, shared in countless ways every day, and his unwavering confidence in the importance of this work make all the difference. She also thanks Virginia Rutter for her cherished friendship; her connections to Neil's legacy and her own wisdom, brilliance, and strength have influenced this work in countless ways. Finally, she is grateful to her daughter, Serena Langdon-Dimidjian, for the joy, wonder, and delight that she discovers in each day, reminding us of all that is possible.

Ruth Herman-Dunn gratefully acknowledges her husband, Christopher Dunn, for his competent advisement and frequent, quick-witted humor. She is thankful to her brother, Edward Herman, for his loving support and lively late-night discussions about BA. Last, she is grateful to her daughter, Ellie, for tolerating frequent refrains of "too busy" and for being a cherished reminder of the importance of each moment.

Foreword

The purpose of *Behavioral Activation for Depression: A Clinician's Guide* is to equip clinicians, regardless of theoretical orientation, with the knowledge they need to utilize behavioral activation (BA) treatment. The authors have successfully accomplished this goal and have produced a great book—one that delineates many behavioral techniques that will be useful to the BA therapist and to his or her patients.

If one thinks of psychological treatments as being on a continuum with regard to how structured they are, BA would be placed toward the structured end of the continuum. Nevertheless, BA treatment must be tailored to the idiosyncratic needs of the patient and requires a substantial amount of flexibility, innovation, and experimentation on the part of the therapist. This is what makes many of the procedures described in the text so useful. I am also impressed with the importance the authors place on the BA therapist's being directive, yet nonjudgmental, and collaborative with clients. The effective BA therapist is not passive.

There are techniques unique to BA (e.g., scheduling of activities), but there are also many techniques that BA shares with other cognitive-behavioral therapies, such as problem solving, treating thoughts as problematic behaviors, and focusing on avoidance and relapse prevention.

In this comprehensive and detailed description of BA, each chapter clearly addresses specific issues, problems, and challenges and explains the kinds of behaviors that are likely to facilitate the therapeutic process. As recognized experts in BA, the authors have a strong commitment to this approach and an excellent record as researchers and clinicians in using these techniques.

The authors briefly mention BA's potential applications for people who also suffer from problems other than depression, such as coping with other medical diseases and caring for elderly individuals with dementia. Clearly there will be important individual differences in how well different clinicians administer the intervention and how well patients respond to this treatment. These are important issues to be addressed by future research.

Although this book is clearly intended to train competent BA therapists and can be effectively utilized by clinicians in their practices, researchers will also find it useful in evaluating the efficacy of various forms of training for therapist skill development. I applaud the authors for providing such a vital resource for our field.

PETER M. LEWINSOHN, PHD
University of Oregon
Eugene, Oregon

Preface

Clinical research and practice are at a crossroads. The history of these areas has been fraught with challenge. Clinicians often have looked askance at researchers, citing concerns that most research studies have little relevance for the daily realities of clinical practice. They raise objections about the restrictions on the types of clients allowed to participate in research studies and the degree to which they resemble actual clients whom clinicians treat. Clinicians also have wondered whether the findings from research studies are relevant to their frequently changing work environments in which they must cope with multiple competing demands to become skilled in empirically supported treatments and to provide services to increasing numbers of clients in less time and often with less funding to do so.

The challenges of coming decades, however, require the strengthening of ties between clinical research and practice. We wrote this book with the practicing psychotherapist in mind. We have been steeped in behavioral activation (BA) through clinical research and practice for the past 10 years, and this book reflects our efforts to integrate these experiences in ways that will be relevant and useful for practicing clinicians.

We highlight the 10 BA principles that guide therapists throughout treatment and describe the core strategies BA therapists use. We include homework forms and handouts that clinicians can use with clients and, throughout the book, we anchor our discussions of clinical strategies in case examples, all of which are based on or inspired by actual clients (disguised suitably to protect confidentiality). We have anticipated the difficulties that therapists might face because we have faced them ourselves. We know that strategies do not always work and that no treatment is a panacea for all problems, and we are continually humbled by our own errors. We have brought that experience to bear on this book and hope therapists will find it practical and inspiring when therapy is going well and when challenges arise. We are committed to bridging the gap between academia and practice. We hope that this book, written for practitioners, scholars, and scientists, increases the likelihood that BA will not only be a subject of further research but that it also will be pursued by many therapists with fidelity in helping their depressed clients build lives that are rich and rewarding.

Contents

BEHAVIORAL ACTIVATION
FOR DEPRESSION

1

Introduction

The Development of Behavioral Activation

The past is never dead. It's not even past.
—WILLIAM FAULKNER (1897–1962)

This book is about behavioral activation (BA), a psychotherapy that has been shown to be an effective treatment for depression and has shown potential for the treatment of other disorders as well. It is written with therapists from many different theoretical orientations in mind. BA is a standalone treatment, but it also is an important part of standard cognitive-behavioral treatment for depression. The principles we present will be useful for therapists who do not typically work from a cognitive-behavior therapy (CBT) framework and find they need greater structure with particular clients. BA has taken several forms over the past four decades and is a focus of renewed interest today following the results of recent clinical research. Yet, behind all research and scientific findings, there is a story. Journal articles present important data, but they do not always tell the story of the ways in which the studies are developed over the course of the actual lives and contributions of those who led the way in the development of these principles and this treatment. This book describes how to put the principles and strategies of BA into practice. Before we get there,

1

we want to share with you the history of the development and study of BA. Enjoy the story.

A Starting Place

There are many possible points in time to start this story. We begin with some memories of our colleague and mentor Neil S. Jacobson, who died in the middle of our work on BA in 1999. For Neil, doing science meant engaging skepticism. As Dimidjian (2000) recalled, Neil "accepted no theory of change, treatment model, or basic tenet or assumption without subjecting it to a rigorous, exacting empiricism" (pg. 1). He often challenged popular opinion and loyalties to particular models. Neil's scientific skepticism was born not only of the enjoyment of a good fight but also of compassion. He wanted to find short-term interventions that provided lasting effects and could be easily disseminated among clinical communities.

Neil also criticized the prevailing treatments of depression as "defect models" because they located the cause of depression as internal deficits within individuals. In contrast, he sought to understand the person in the full context of the treatment of depression and encouraged us to look outside the individual in our effort to understand and treat depression. It was his supposition that the secret to alleviating depression lay in changing the conditions in people's lives. In these ways, then, we begin our story of BA with skepticism and compassion, two essential ingredients for science to advance clinical change.

What Are the Active Ingredients of Therapy for Depression?

The theory behind BA owes its development to work that has been done over the past three decades on understanding and alleviating depression. Research on therapies for depression has focused most heavily on cognitive therapy (CT) for depression. Developed by Aaron T. Beck and his associates, CT is based on the assumption that the way people *think* about situations in their lives influences how they feel and what they do. When people are depressed, they exhibit problematic ways of thinking that increase their depression. CT focuses on how to help people identify such depressive thoughts and beliefs, evaluate how these thoughts impact them, and make changes in such thinking patterns. The primary hypothesis in CT is that when people think more realistically they will feel better. The strategies used in CT are multifaceted and include three primary categories: behavioral strategies designed to change how people act in situations, cognitive strategies designed to change how people think about specific situations, and cognitive strategies designed to change the enduring central beliefs that people have about themselves, their future, and the world. The CT approach places particular importance on cognitive strategies. Although behavioral strategies are emphasized in the treatment of more severely depressed individuals, the goal of moving to cognitive change strategies is clear in CT. Beck and colleagues described the use of behavioral strategies in the seminal treatment manual for CT, explaining, "The ultimate aim of these techniques in cognitive therapy is to produce change in the negative attitudes" (Beck, Rush, Shaw, & Emery, 1979, p. 118).

Many studies have attested to the efficacy of CT, including some recent rigorous clinical trials (DeRubeis et al., 2005; Hollon et al., 2005). These studies, however, did not address some important questions. It seemed pretty clear that CT did work, but do we really know *how* it worked? What are the active ingredients of CT? Are all the strategies of CT needed to produce positive outcomes? Could the behavioral strategies of CT alone account for the success of cognitive therapy?

A series of studies have tried to address these questions. Zeiss, Lewinsohn, and Muñoz (1979) conducted one of the earliest studies, finding that depressed participants improved regardless of the specific components of the treatment. Their group of depressed outpatients received either cognitive restructuring, interpersonal skills training, or pleasant events scheduling. All of the treatments were successful in eliminating depression. Zettle and Rains (1989) compared three group therapies: complete cognitive therapy, partial cognitive therapy, and a contextual approach referred to as comprehensive distancing. All groups showed significant and equal reductions in depression over the 12-week treatment and 2-month follow-up. In 1989, Scogin, Jamison, and Gochneaur found that cognitively focused bibliotherapy and behaviorally based bibliotherapy were both superior to control conditions, but both interventions were of equal efficacy.

Perhaps the most widely influential of studies addressing the active ingredients of CT is the component analysis study published in 1996 by Jacobson and colleagues (Jacobson et al., 1996). In this type of study, the different components of a treatment are isolated and compared to one another in an aim to identify which parts of the treatment are causally active. Some 150 depressed adults enrolled in this component analysis study were randomly assigned to one of three treatments: (1) the behavioral activation component, (2) the behavioral activation plus cognitive restructuring of automatic thoughts component, or (3) the full cognitive therapy package, consisting of behavioral activation, cognitive restructuring of automatic thoughts, and cognitive restructuring of core beliefs.

The first condition (BA) allowed therapists to use the behavioral strategies such as activity scheduling, mastery/pleasure ratings, and graded task assignments, strategies we describe in much more detail in subsequent chapters. In the second condition (BA plus automatic thought restructuring), therapists could use the behavioral strategies and cognitive strategies designed to change how one thinks in specific situations. In the third condition, therapists could use any of the strategies used in the other conditions, and they could also work on changing core beliefs about the self, world, and future—that is, the full range of CT strategies as outlined in Beck et al. (1979) and subsequent treatment manuals (e.g., J. S. Beck, 1995).

The same therapists provided all of the treatments and, in fact, were strongly in favor of the full CT approach. They used cognitive conceptualizations for clients assigned to all of the treatment conditions and generally believed that utilizing the BA component solely was akin to doing therapy with one hand tied behind their backs. They felt discouraged when their patients were randomly assigned to the BA component condition, and their reactions paralleled those of most people in the field—namely, that participants in the BA (only) condition would show poorer outcomes.

What happened, though, surprised many! There were no significant differences among the three treatments, either in the acute treatment of depression or in the prevention of relapse across a 2-year follow-up (Jacobson et al., 1996; Gortner, Gollan, Dobson, & Jacobson, 1998). Results obtained from the BA component condition were comparable to those from the full cognitive therapy program. This finding caused quite a stir, and numerous notes of caution were raised. Some rejected the findings, suggesting that the therapy had not been done properly and that the substandard quality of CT explained the pattern of findings (Jacobson & Gortner, 2000). Others were intrigued by the findings but believed that replicating them in another study was necessary.

The authors of the component analysis study thought there was much of value in the critiques and agreed that it was necessary to seek replication and to do so in a way that ensured the CT was performed as competently as possible. The results of the component analysis study galvanized our research group around some central questions as we continued to pursue this work. We began to wonder whether purely behavioral approaches had been overlooked in recent decades. Was the whole field missing something important that behavioral approaches might be able to offer in the treatment of depression?

Back to Behavioral Roots

The questions raised by the component analysis study spurred us to return to the literature. We started reading research studies that addressed behavioral approaches to depression. In some cases, these studies had been published decades ago. We requested papers from old journals in the libraries and dusted off old books from our shelves. As we read this literature, our thinking about BA evolved. We began to develop the basis for a behavioral treatment that was defined in its own right, not exclusively by the proscription of cognitive interventions as it had been in the component analysis study (Jacobson, Martell, & Dimidjian, 2001; Martell, Addis, & Jacobson, 2001).

As interest in BA for depression was revitalized by the component analysis study, the development of BA was also grounded in a long tradition of behavioral theory and research, much of which we realized had gone largely unnoticed in recent decades. In particular, BA builds on the foundation of the work of four important early pioneers: Charles B. Ferster, Peter M. Lewinsohn, Lynn P. Rehm, and Aaron T. Beck. While Ferster focused on the theory underlying the behavioral analysis of depression, Lewinsohn extended the theory and developed behavioral treatment methods for depression, Rehm emphasized the importance of reinforcement in the treatment of depression, and Beck made behavioral activation available to a larger clinical audience by including it as an integral part of CT for depression. We discuss the contributions and influence of these fore-fathers of BA next.

Charles B. Ferster

Ferster (1973) prostulated that a decrease in certain types of activity and an increase in other types characterized depression. Ferster focused in particular on the increase in escape and avoidance behaviors and as a result suggested that depressed persons received fewer rewards from their activities. He proposed a few reasons why this might be the case. First, he suggested that depressed people might not engage in productive activities frequently enough, which lessens the effectiveness of the reinforcement of such activities. Second, he suggested that depressed individuals might engage in behavior that was motivated by attempts to escape from aversive feelings, which "prevented positively reinforced behavior" (p. 859). Thus, depressed people's behavior may be controlled primarily by negative reinforcement as opposed to positive reinforcement. In other words, actions serve the purpose of reducing an aversive state rather than allowing the person to engage the environment in such a way that the behavior is naturally rewarded and positively reinforced.

All behavior occurs in a particular context, and behavior is reinforced by its consequences. These are the *contingencies* of behavior. Ferster (1973) emphasized the ways in which a depressed client's limited interactions with his or her environment can result in a diminished ability to learn from contingencies. The focus on one's internal state of deprivation as opposed to a focus on observing one's environment, according to Ferster, is "a serious impediment to an improvement of the depressed person's view of the world. The depressed person may not be able to emit enough potentially reinforceable behavior to discover the differential reaction of the environment, depending on the kind of performance that is emitted" (p. 39).

As we readily acknowledge, the current BA model is grounded in many of Ferster's early ideas. His work provided a sound behavior-analytic framework for looking at the *function* of behavior rather than just its form. BA was intended as a flexible treatment tailored to each individual client. The BA model does not assume that any particular class of behavior is necessarily reinforcing for a client, such as increasing pleasant events. Rather, the BA model uses functional analysis (discussed throughout this book) to increase behaviors that have the greatest potential to help the client interact with an environment and that provide consequences that will positively reinforce antidepressant behavior. The emphasis on the function over the form of behavior remains a major contribution of the early work of Ferster to BA.

Peter M. Lewinsohn

Lewinsohn's theory of depression was consistent with many of the elements proposed by Ferster. Lewinsohn highlighted the importance of the lack of positive reinforcement in depressed patients' lives. Specifically, he conceptualized depression as a result of a lack, or low rate, of "response-contingent" positive reinforcement (Lewinsohn, 1974). Response contingent means that reinforcement is dependent on the individual's actions. For example, if a person in a relationship tries to make conversation and the partner ignores the attempt (does not provide response-contingent positive reinforcement) or rebuffs it as "clingy" (punishes), the individual will eventually stop making attempts at conversing with the partner and feel sad about the relationship. It follows that this person is less likely to make conversation over time, and, in other words, conversation behavior may become extinguished. This lack of positive reinforcement is hypothesized to limit behaviors that typically result in rewards from individuals' lives, which can cause or maintains dysphoria.

Lewinsohn (1974) also pointed out that low rates of response-contingent positive reinforcement can operate in contexts that may seem surprising; for instance, he explained that job promotions can lead to *loss* of social reinforcement (e.g., losing peers in the transition to a managerial position) or that achieving a goal for which one has worked long and hard (e.g., attaining an academic degree) may turn out to be a weak reinforcer for the individual. He explained, "It is not the absolute amount of attention or other 'goodies' received that is critical but the fact that the environment provides consequences sufficient to maintain the individual's behavior" (p. 180). Clearly, Lewinsohn believed that the subjective experience of environmental rewards trumps their face value in determining their subsequent impact on behavior and mood.

Lewinsohn and colleagues eventually revised their model to explain how negative life events affect some people and not others. Lewinsohn, Hoberman, Teri, and Hautzinger (1985) suggest that negative life events decrease the likelihood of adaptive behaviors for vulnerable individuals who may lack the skills for coping with the events. These disruptions and the accompanying dysphoric mood lead to the individual's becoming excessively self-focused and self-critical. There is also a decrease in motivation, and the vulnerable individual withdraws from social contacts. Thus, there is a downward spiral into further depression as the individual deactivates in response to the disruption.

In these ways, Lewinsohn's work contributed the importance of understanding the contingencies in the individual client's life. Lewinsohn and Libet (1972) found that depressed individuals might be more vulnerable to the ups and downs of everyday life. Depressed individuals also respond more to an aversive stimulus than do nondepressed individuals. Just as some people have a lower tolerance for physical pain and will become highly distressed at a twisted ankle while others will continue to walk around with the same level of injury, depressed individuals are likely to be more reactive to the pain of life—emotional as well as physical—than those who are not depressed. Lewinsohn (1974) suggested that desensitization to aversive situations might be a useful therapeutic tool.

Importantly, Lewinsohn and colleagues (Lewinsohn, 1974; Lewinsohn, Biglan, & Zeiss, 1976) were the first to incorporate activity scheduling into the behavioral treatment they developed for depression. In this approach, they assessed the frequency and range of pleasant events in a client's life. They developed activity schedules, breaking the week into hourly segments, and asked clients to plan pleasant activities in their week. Over time, clients increased their activity and engaged in behaviors that they either wished to do or had once done but had stopped since becoming depressed. Lewinsohn and colleagues also developed a self-report measure, the Pleasant Events Schedule (PES), to assess pleasant events occurring in an individual's life over the past month (Lewinsohn & Graf, 1973; Lewinsohn & Libet, 1972; MacPhillamy & Lewinsohn, 1982). The PES lists 320 events for which individuals are asked to rate the frequency and the degree to which each event was "pleasant, enjoyable, or rewarding."

Lewinsohn's work has profoundly influenced the BA approach that we describe in this book. His research on both behavioral models of depression and behavioral interventions established the foundations on which the current BA approach was built. Specifically, his emphasis on the importance of understanding reinforcement contingencies has informed our emphasis on the use of behavioral assessment to guide treatment planning and targeting. A general aim of BA is to help the client to activate in ways that will increase the likelihood that his or her behavior will be positively reinforced. Lewinsohn's focus ✓ on aversive control has also shaped our emphasis on helping clients to take action and solve problems in order to live richer lives, even at times in the midst of negative feelings. His understanding of the excessive self-focus of depressed individuals informs our approach to treating the process and function of depressive rumination. Finally, the strategies he used clinically, such as monitoring weekly activities and scheduling ongoing activities, are the mainstays of BA practice and procedures.

Lynn P. Rehm

While Rehm's model of depression included components that are considered more cognitive, such as selective attention to negative events (Fuchs & Rehm, 1977), it was also distinctly behavioral. Rehm (1977) emphasized the importance of reinforcement in depression and proposed a self-control model of depression and therapy for depression. Rehm's model used Kanfer's (1970) definition of self-control as "those processes by which an individual alters the probability of a response in the relative absence of immediate external supports" (Rehm, 1977, p. 790). The self-control model postulates a feedback loop consisting of self-monitoring, self-evaluation, and self-reinforcement. An example of self-monitoring would be a student's keeping track of her grade-point average. Self-evaluation is a comparison between an estimate of performance and an internal standard. Stated simply, the student has observed that her grade-point average has been a 4.0 and may evaluate a grade of 3.5 as failure because it doesn't meet her standard. If she typically downloads a few favorite songs when she gets a 4.0, she may not reward herself in the same way for the 3.5. Comparisons of one's behavior, however, are predicated on the attribution that the cause of a behavior is internal, that is, "I did not work hard enough." A perception of internal control is required in order for one to attempt self-control of behavior, that is, "I can do better than this." Also, one must be able to reinforce oneself for behavior that does not meet with immediately rewarding consequences—for example, the student rewards herself by downloading music, although the longer-term consequences of getting high grades is that she graduates with honors and increases her chances of future success.

According to this model, depression is accounted for by deficits in self-control behavior, specifically in "(1) selective monitoring of negative events; (2) selective monitoring of immediate as opposed to delayed consequences of behavior; (3) stringent self-evaluative criteria; (4) inaccurate attributions of responsibility; (5) insufficient self-reward; and (6) excessive self-punishment" (Rehm, 1977, p. 795). Depressed persons selectively attend to negative feedback, and their behavior elicits immediate reinforcement at the expense of important delayed reinforcement. When people are depressed, they make external attributions of causality and set stringent standards for self-evaluation. Finally, according to the self-control model, depression is characterized by relatively low rates of self-reinforcement and relatively high rates of self-punishment. The depressed individual is more susceptible to mood fluctuations occasioned by external events rather than self-reward to supplement and maintain behavior regardless of external environmental events. Deficits in self-reinforcement result in a reduction of sustained effort and a tendency to engage in behavior that is *immediately* reinforced. Such deficits in sustained effort and responses to immediate consequences may encourage high frequencies of behaviors that function as avoidance behaviors, which are discussed at length in later chapters. Furthermore, excessive self-punishment may result in unduly inhibited thoughts, speech, or actions, or in excessively negative self-statements and evaluations. Rehm's work has been influential in extending the understanding of the nature of reinforcement and the need to look at the client's predilection to benefit from short-term (versus long-term) rewards.

Aaron T. Beck

In 1979, Beck and colleagues published *Cognitive Therapy of Depression*. This text and its dissemination profoundly changed the landscape of mental health service delivery for depression. The empirical support for cognitive therapy and cognitive-behavioral therapies for depression has led to CBTs becoming one of the strongest empirically supported treatments for depression. In essence, it is the gold standard of brief treatment for depression. In his cognitive therapy approach, Beck integrated BA strategies in a larger cognitive framework. Although this cognitive-behavioral approach eclipsed the purely behavioral approaches that preceded it, it also helped to formalize core BA strategies and make them widely available. In this way, Beck promoted the value of BA more than many pure behaviorists.

Beck's model of cognitive therapy for depression specifies that treatment should begin with activation—particularly with more seriously depressed clients—prior to monitoring and modifying specific beliefs. Moreover, behavioral strategies are optimally integrated throughout treatment as a key means of exploring and evaluating cognition.

One of the primary contributions of CT to behavioral strategies includes the ways in which CT has formalized a method for activity monitoring and scheduling. In CT, clients record activities on an activity schedule and are asked to record whether the activity gave them a sense of pleasure or mastery (accomplishment). Therapists assist clients in developing a rating scale for mastery and pleasure. J. S. Beck (1995) suggests having clients develop a 0–10 rating scale, identifying specific behaviors that would give them a sense of accomplishment or pleasure at the various poles of the scale and along the continuum. Thus, the client can use his or her scale as a guide for rating how much mastery or pleasure an activity allowed. For example, a client may select "brushing my teeth" as providing zero sense of accomplishment, "making the bed" may be rated as a "5," and "mowing the backyard" as a "10" on his or her individualized scale. Similar anchors for pleasure may be generated. Using this as a guideline, when the client engages in an activity such as dusting furniture in the den, he or she can compare dusting to the three tasks on the scale and determine if it is closer to making the bed (a "5") or mowing the backyard (a "10") and rate it accordingly.

Behavioral techniques in CT always serve the ultimate goal of changing how people think since belief change is considered to be essential for lasting improvement in behavioral or emotional problems. In contrast, this is a distinct difference in BA, where activity is encouraged hopefully to bring the client into contact with positive reinforcers that will maintain or increase further antidepressant activity. Both CT and BA ask clients to engage in behavioral experiments. However, in BA the client is asked to conduct experiments to evaluate the outcome, impact on mood, impact on goals, and so forth. In CT, clients are asked to conduct "experiments" in order to test their depressive assumptions and expectations. Despite the differences, the development of CT provided an essential foundation for the development of the current model of BA. In addition to the overlap in specific strategies, as noted above, BA also adopts an emphasis on structuring sessions that is characteristic of CT. Nonbehavioral psychotherapists are more likely to make use of activation strategies, thanks to the work of Aaron T. Beck and his associates. This is all to the benefit of depressed clients, for whom simple activation procedures appear to be a necessary treatment for reduction of symptoms.

The Empirical Evidence Base for BA

The contemporary model of BA was put to a rigorous test in a clinical trial at the University of Washington (the Seattle study). This study was important because it addressed some of the major limitations of the earlier component analysis study. It compared BA not only to CT but also to antidepressant medication. Previous research had suggested that psychotherapy (specifically CT) was not efficacious among patients with moderate to severe major depression (Elkin et al., 1989). Treatment guidelines had been issued suggesting that, although less severely depressed patients may benefit from psychotherapy, moderately to severely depressed patients required antidepressant medication for successful treatment (American Psychiatric Association Workgroup on Major Depressive Disorder, 2000). Thus, the study compared BA to the most widely studied psychotherapy, CT, and the current standard of care, pharmacotherapy. Experts in each of the treatment modalities collaborated on the study, ensuring that highly respected cognitive therapists and pharmacotherapists were involved in the planning, execution, and analysis of the study. Throughout the study, these advocates for each treatment were charged with overseeing the quality with which their preferred treatment was being implemented.

Specifically, BA was compared to CT and to antidepressant

medication (paroxetine) in the context of a placebo-controlled trial with 241 depressed adults. The results of this study were provocative. The analysis focused on how the treatments compared between the two groups of interest: the less and more severely depressed patients. The acute outcomes of patients who received BA were comparable to those who received antidepressant medication, even among more severely depressed patients. Patients assigned to BA tended to stay in treatment longer than those assigned to pharmacotherapy. BA was also superior to CT in the acute treatment of more severely depressed patients. There were no differences among treatments for the less severely depressed patients. Longer-term follow-up data showed indications that the benefits of BA were as enduring as those of CT in helping patients prevent relapse or future episodes of depression. Participants who had responded to pharmacotherapy relapsed at greater rates when withdrawn from their medications than participants who had prior BA or CT (Dimidjian et al., 2006; Dobson et al., 2008).

Like all studies, the Seattle study was not without its limitations. In retrospect, we might have prescribed the antidepressant medications in a different way to help people stay in treatment longer. We also would have enrolled more patients so that we could have had a larger sample to adequately run all of the statistical analyses we preferred. And, like any study, the findings need to be replicated at other places by other people. There are important questions that we are pursuing with our current research. In this way, the story of BA, with which we started, is ongoing even today. Although no one study can answer all the important research questions, we did learn from the Seattle study that BA has promise in the treatment of depression. Moreover, our excitement about the results is bolstered by a number of other lines of converging results.

Related Activation Treatments for Depression

The theory and conceptualization of BA are finding support in other related activation-based interventions for depression. Many of the central concepts in BA, such as activation, scheduling activities, and engaging in problem solving rather than passive ruminating, are critical to these related approaches as well. The findings supporting these related approaches have influenced our thinking about BA and have provided independent support for the central tenets of the BA approach to depression.

Brief Behavioral Activation Treatment for Depression

During the time that the Seattle study was being conducted, Carl Lejuez and colleagues (Lejuez, Hopko, LePage, Hopko, & McNeil, 2001) conducted a similar line of research into what they referred to as behavioral activation treatment for depression (BATD) independent of the research being done in Washington. In several small studies they have also found that activating depressed clients is an effective treatment for depressed inpatients (Hopko, Lejuez, LePage, Hopko, & McNeil, 2003), depressed cancer patients (Hopko, Bell, Armento, Hunt, & Lejuez, 2005), and clients with comorbid depression and anxiety (Hopko, Lejuez, & Hopko, 2004). These researchers have utilized a brief form of activation that consists exclusively of activity monitoring and scheduling. Clients are asked to develop a list of activity goals for the week and then to note on each day whether they attempted the activity or not and if they achieved their goal for that activity. This approach is highly compatible with BA and again provides a converging line of evidence for the importance of activating depressed clients.

Problem-Solving Therapy

Problem solving is a mainstay of BA and has a history of evidence as a treatment for depression (Gotlib & Asarnow, 1979; Nezu, 1987). The problem-solving approaches, for the most part, consider the individual client, define the problems experienced by the client, set targets for treatment, and then implement therapeutic techniques that have empirical support in the treatment of various problems or skill deficits (Biglan & Dow, 1981). Problem-solving therapy has been shown to be an efficacious treatment for depression in primary care settings as well and can be conducted by trained psychiatrists, psychiatric nurses, or general practitioners (Mynors-Wallis, Gath, Davies, Gray, & Barbour, 1997).

Similarities to Newer Behavior Therapies

BA has been developed during a time when cognitive-behavioral therapies are being transformed. Interest in more purely behavioral approaches is increasing, and thoughts are being dealt with in different ways than the original cognitive therapies proposed by Beck and others. Several new therapies have a focus that is very consistent with BA. The accumulating evidence for these approaches adds to the weight of data suggesting that activation is a key ingredient in the clinical change process and that BA represents part of a larger shift back to behavioral roots that have been underemphasized in the past two decades.

Dialectical behavior therapy (DBT) was developed for the treatment of highly suicidal clients diagnosed with borderline personality disorder (Linehan, 1993). The therapy consists of a number of component skills that are taught to clients to assist them in regulating their moods. One of the core skills utilized in DBT is referred to as "opposite action," in which clients are taught to act in ways that are opposite to the action urges of emotions that they want to change. For example, a person who feels angry at a slow parking garage attendant and has a strong desire to curse may act in an opposite manner, smiling and saying in a warm and friendly tone, "Thank you, have a great day." BA, in many ways, is "opposite action" for depression. The urge in depression is often not to act, or to escape or avoid; activating goes against that urge.

Acceptance and commitment therapy (ACT), developed by Hayes and colleagues, is another approach with accumulating support that shares similar treatment targets to BA (Hayes, Luoma, Bond, Masuda, & Lillis, 2006; Hayes, Strosahl, & Wilson, 1999). Specifically, ACT emphasizes that clients break patterns of experiential avoidance and make a commitment to action that will help them attain a life that they value. This attention to values was underemphasized when we wrote the original manual for BA (Martell et al., 2001), but is a useful idea to incorporate when treating clients. In an early version of ACT, Zettle and Rains (1987) evaluated comprehensive distancing (CD) versus CT. CD focused on letting go of efforts to change negative thoughts and acting effectively even in the presence of negative thoughts. Zettle and Rains (1987) reported evidence of promise for CD.

David H. Barlow, considered one of the most influential psychologists of the late 20th century, has noted similarities in treatments across several disorders (Barlow, Allen, & Choate, 2004). Barlow and colleagues (2004) noted that a common strategy that has been utilized in a number of treatments is to modify action tendencies in response to emotional dysregulation. They state:

In modifying the behavioral action tendencies driven by fundamental emotions, the first step is to provoke the emotions in so far as possible.... Adopting strategies that encourage experience of the emotion without engaging in the associated action tendencies (accepting the emotion) is a very basic strategy in this regard. When applied to specific disorders, emotional and behavioral activation, especially in situational context, becomes a particularly powerful tool. (pp. 223–224)

Barlow and colleagues emphasize the value of a "unified" approach to the treatment of mood and anxiety problems. It is possible that BA may be a core ingredient of a range of efficacious treatments and, as such, may have value as a transdiagnostic approach. Such possibilities, however, are purely speculative at this time and require rigorous research to examine the potential promise and limitations of BA across a range of presenting problems.

Summary

The history of BA is ongoing. The earlier development of behavioral and cognitive-behavioral treatments for depression continues to inform current research. Our return to the behavioral basics to develop a straightforward treatment for depression that acknowledges the problematic lives with which many depressed people struggle has been part of a wider resurgence of behavioral treatments. BA is consistent with other newly developed behavioral interventions as the fields of behavior therapy and CBT continue to evolve. Having reviewed the story of how BA developed, the evidence that supports its use, and how it fits into the grand scheme of contemporary behavior therapy, we are now ready to turn to the core principles and strategies of BA.

2

The Core Principles
of Behavioral Activation

[People] acquire a particular quality by constantly acting
a particular way.... You become just by performing just
actions, temperate by performing temperate actions, brave by
performing brave actions.
—ARISTOTLE (384 B.C.–322 B.C.)

Alicia dreaded getting out of bed every morning since being laid off from her programming job. She knew that layoffs were common, but she also blamed herself for having challenged her boss too many times and speaking out of turn at meetings. With her unemployment benefits as her only income, it was very difficult in the beginning to make ends meet. Living on such a small amount of money required her to sell her condominium and rent a smaller apartment. Alicia believed that she would have more energy and hope once she found the right job. Such a job was not forthcoming, however. She looked for 8 months for another programming position before settling on a temporary job updating websites for a small company. The position did not pay well, and she was thoroughly bored by the tasks. Her supervisor seemed to have little interest in Alicia's work or schedule, and there was little consequence when Alicia arrived at work as much as 2 hours late; so, she stayed in bed.

The drudgery of her work was not the only problem. She also was experiencing a great deal of worry and anxiety. She had experienced such feelings before being laid off; in fact, she occasionally had missed work before after having lost sleep worrying through much of the night. She worried more nights than not, and her worries focused on how badly she felt and about whether she would make ends meet and succeed in life. Most frequently, however, she worried about how much her moods undermined her relationships.

Elements of Alicia's case are likely familiar to most readers who have worked with depressed clients. We use it throughout the book to illustrate key points about BA and to highlight how BA conceptualization and interventions work. As the description of Alicia's case proceeds, you can follow the general course of her treatment with her BA therapist.

Changes in Alicia's life multiplied and her mood worsened as she began to disengage from people and activities that used to bring pleasure and stimulation to her life. Since moving into the smaller apartment, Alicia also had stopped inviting any of her friends to visit. She was embarrassed by the size of the unit and the cheap construction of the building. Her neighborhood was safe but in an undesirable section of town that she and her friends used to snicker at and referred to as "the runway" because it was near the airport. She had lived in this same neighborhood for a year after finishing college, never dreaming she would go backward in her life, returning to the small, cheerless dwellings that looked like converted motels. So, she did not invite her friends over and rarely visited them, because she dreaded the inevitable conversation about employment. Feeling envy over their relative good fortune also felt bad; so, it was easier for her to avoid the contact altogether. Unfortunately, a few of her friends had taken Alicia's distance personally after she cancelled on three or four events; they no longer called her. She missed them but could not muster the nerve to call and explain her behavior.

Alicia found the apparent rejection by her friends intolerable because she had a long history of family problems, which ultimately led to her mothers' kicking her out of the house 2 months after her 17th birthday. She went to live with friends and did not talk to her mother for over 3 years. She described this as a very sad and "nerve-wracking" time of her life.

While there are many roads to depression, readers may also find the types of things that have happened to Alicia common in the lives of their depressed clients. Alicia had, indeed, become depressed and met criteria for a major depressive disorder. Her medical doctor suggested that she take an antidepressant medication to treat her depression and anxiety. "Great. Now I'm crazy as well as broke," she thought. When she vehemently refused to take "crazy drugs," her doctor asked her to at least have a few visits with a psychotherapist. Without health insurance, the cost of any treatment seemed prohibitive. Alicia agreed to meet a therapist, but only for a few visits. The doctor referred her to someone known for her skill at brief interventions.

Alicia was surprised by the way the therapist interacted with her in the first session. She had expected the woman to sit back quietly and nod as she poured out her life story. The therapist, Beth, instead asked about her sleep and eating habits, her mood, level of enjoyment of activities, use of alcohol or drugs, and social interactions. Beth also focused on how life was prior to Alicia's job crisis. What were Alicia's plans for her life? What had she expected things to be like at this time?

Answering such questions was painful. Alicia had expected to sell her condo and buy a house, not to sell her condo and rent a lousy apartment. She thought she might be dating someone rather than barely holding onto a handful of friends who remained very committed to her. When Beth pointed out to her how unrewarding her life had become, Alicia could not agree more. Beth also explained that the feelings of sadness, fatigue, and hopelessness were natural and often experienced when life is unrewarding. She explained that these feelings often followed periods of anxiety and worry and that they certainly were understandable after losing a good job. Beth also said that staying in bed actually made sense when one felt these feelings. Alicia was curious. She often told herself (and heard in the advice shared by her family members) that her behavior made no sense at all. If she was having a hard time, she asked herself, why not just try a little harder instead of staying in bed all morning? Getting a new job could not be that hard, she said to herself—countless times a day.

Beth proposed BA as the plan of treatment. "The goal is to get you re-engaged in the activities that once brought pleasure and satisfaction to you, even though the circumstances of your life have changed," she explained. "This may also help in problem solving the worrisome situations you find yourself losing sleep over." Alicia thought, "I can't imagine feeling much pleasure or satisfaction about anything, and certainly can't imagine not worrying about it all." When Beth asked if she was willing to try six sessions to evaluate whether this approach proved helpful prior to committing to a longer course of therapy, Alicia concluded that she had nothing to lose by trying.

Introduction

Alicia's therapist, Beth, introduced the basic concepts of behavior therapy for depression. BA interventions have been a core component of behavioral and cognitive-behavioral treatments for depression for decades. In recent years, BA has gained increasing attention as a stand-alone treatment for depression. What accounts for this rising interest in BA? As we discussed in Chapter 1, there are two likely explanations. First, the principles underlying BA are simple, and the treatment procedures used in BA are straightforward. Second, the empirical studies conducted to date suggest that BA works.

This book is designed to give you the information you need to implement BA with the depressed clients that you treat. Whereas other published manuals address the theoretical background and conceptual model of BA (Martell et al., 2001), we focus here on identifying the core principles and putting them into practice. We first discuss how a BA therapist structures therapy and the general style of a BA therapist. We then discuss how to identify primary treatment targets in BA through the use of behavioral assessment and the development of a case conceptualization. Next, we turn to the primary treatment procedures relevant to increasing activation, decreasing avoidance, and addressing ruminative thinking. Our goal is to provide a comprehensive guide to the variety of techniques that help clients get active and engaged in their lives.

We will discuss these techniques in the context of our work with specific clients in research studies and in real-world clinical settings. We also draw on the history of behavior therapy and the scientific support from clinical research and other related areas of psychology to orient you to the evidence base for this treatment. Having a solid knowledge of this evidence can help you, as scientists and practitioners, to understand and explain the treatment to the clients you treat. Ultimately, we hope this book will help you conceptualize the problems of the clients you see, develop treatment plans, and implement strategies in as effective a fashion as possible.

What Is BA for Depression?

BA is a brief structured treatment for depression that aims to activate clients in specific ways that will increase rewarding experiences in their lives. All of the techniques of BA are used in the service of the fundamental goal of increasing activation and engagement in one's world. Toward this end, BA also focuses on processes that inhibit activation, such as escape and avoidance behaviors. BA is based on the premise that problems in vulnerable individuals' lives reduce their ability to experience positive reward from their environments, leading to the symptoms and behaviors that we classify as depression. In order to alleviate depression, BA assumes clients must be assisted in engaging in behavior that they will ultimately find pleasurable or productive, or that will improve their life situations in such a way as to provide greater rewards. Sessions in BA are action-oriented and focused on problem solving. In fact, the bulk of the work in therapy happens outside of the therapist's office. Each week, therapists and clients work together to develop activation assignments to be completed between sessions and to troubleshoot any barriers to activation that may arise.

Within this structured framework, BA is highly individualized. Early in therapy, the client and therapist work together to identify behavior patterns related to depression. These patterns can vary substantially between clients. In this book, you will learn how to identify these patterns and use this understanding to develop effective activation plans accordingly. For example, some clients spend time involved in passive behaviors, such as sleeping excessively, watching television, or drinking, which help them to dull negative feelings. Other clients are very active and have no difficulty completing daily tasks; yet, they find themselves caught in an endless cycle of ruminative thinking and experience little pleasure in the activities in which they are involved. Based on an analysis of particular patterns of behavior, a select number of treatment targets are identified; subsequent sessions focus on the ongoing process of changing behavior in these areas.

Because BA is tailored to the individual needs of each client, a wide range of treatment targets can be addressed. For example, a successful course of BA with one man aimed to increase the time that he spent with his children and his degree of engagement when he was with them. His focus of activation thus was structuring his time around parenting and learning to focus his attention away from ruminative thoughts and toward the experience of fatherhood. A woman who sought treatment with BA was helped to learn to allow negative feelings to be present and specifically to grieve a lost relationship that was very important to her. Her activation, thus, was learning to approach her sadness and take steps toward reinitiating old and building new relationships in her life. Another client began to take steps toward finding a new job through updating her résumé, calling former colleagues to ask about job leads, and practicing job interviews. During this time, she also started a schedule of exercising and woke up at a consistent time each day.

The 10 Core Principles of BA

Clearly, there are many ways in which clients can benefit from BA. What unifies these different courses of treatment, however, is a consistent focus on getting active and engaged in one's life. Therapy focuses on figuring out what patterns are maintaining depression and what areas of change will likely improve a client's mood, and then repeatedly and persistently making changes in these areas. Within this basic structure, the BA therapist is guided by a set of simple principles (see Table 2.1).

Principle 1: The key to changing how people feel is helping them change what they do.

Typically, people wait to act until they feel an inner compulsion, or at least inclination, to do something specific. When given free choice on a weekend, a person goes to a movie because he or she feels like it, watches television because he or she isn't motivated to do anything else, or climbs a mountain because he or she feels adventurous. We refer to this as acting from the "inside-out" because the motivation to engage in activity originates from inside. Most of our daily routines, however, include activities for which there is little

TABLE 2.1. The 10 Core Principles of Behavioral Activation

Principle 1: The key to changing how people feel is helping them change what they do.

Principle 2: Changes in life can lead to depression, and short-term coping strategies may keep people stuck over time.

Principle 3: The clues to figuring out what will be antidepressant for a particular client lie in what precedes and follows the client's important behaviors.

Principle 4: Structure and schedule activities that follow a plan, not a mood.

Principle 5: Change will be easier when starting small.

Principle 6: Emphasize activities that are naturally reinforcing.

Principle 7: Act as a coach.

Principle 8: Emphasize a problem-solving empirical approach, and recognize that all results are useful.

Principle 9: Don't just talk, do!

Principle 10: Troubleshoot possible and actual barriers to activation.

From *Behavioral Activation for Depression: A Clinician's Guide* by Christopher R. Martell, Sona Dimidjian, and Ruth Herman-Dunn. Copyright 2010 by The Guilford Press. Permission to photocopy this table is granted to purchasers of this book for personal use only (see copyright page for details). Purchasers may download a larger version of this table from the book's page on The Guilford Press website.

choice, such as going to work every morning or taking care of family or household responsibilities. When people are not depressed, they typically do these tasks regardless of whether they feel like it or not. On a cold, dreary morning, for example, one may feel no motivation to get dressed and go to work, but one does the necessary tasks and gets to work. Once there, one often finds that a sense of interest and accomplishment follows. We refer to this as acting from the "outside-in": engage in an activity, and the feelings follow (Martell et al., 2001). When presenting this idea at a recent workshop, one participant described it as the "field of dreams" approach to change: build a life that is rich and rewarding, and the positive feelings will come.

> *Principle 2:* Changes in life can lead to depression, and short-term coping strategies may keep people stuck over time.

BA is based on certain assumptions about what keeps people stuck in depression and what can help people move in the direction of more satisfying and rewarding lives. Specifically, in BA, we focus on the specific ways that life events (ranging from daily hassles and minor ongoing stressors to major life changes) can lead to decreases in positive reinforcement or increases in punishment that can result in general dysphoria and withdrawal from normal activities. These problems can be considered the primary problems in the client's life. Poor living conditions, unhappy relationships, bad jobs, and ongoing disappointments are all examples of the kinds of problems that can result in the primary problem of low levels of positive reinforcement or high levels of punishment. What often happens for people, however, is that they respond to these primary problems with behaviors that keep them stuck. As an individual stops engaging in activities that were once pleasurable, engages in escape or avoidance behaviors, or responds mostly to behaviors that bring immediate relief from annoyance despite future adverse consequences, such actions become secondary problems in and of themselves (Jacobson et al., 2001; Martell et al., 2001). It is easy to get caught in a continual cycle of feeling down, pulling away from one's world and doing less, and as a consequence feeling more down. Depression is thus maintained as people avoid potential sources of antidepressant reinforcement in their lives because such contact is experienced by them as too challenging or threatening in the short term. Such avoidance provides short-term relief but maintains depression over the long term, both because rewards are not experienced and because stressors in life become worse over time.

Early in therapy, BA therapists present a conceptualization of depression to clients utilizing Principle 2. Some clients will have preconceptions and questions about their depression based on other explanations and information they have heard. Therapists may keep in mind that the principles of BA are not assumed to replace other models of depression, such as cognitive, interpersonal, or biological models. There are solid clinical research studies that support treatments based on such models (e.g., Hollon, Thase, & Markowitz, 2002), and it is prudent for the BA therapist to be informed about such approaches in order to discuss them with clients. The BA conceptualization and treatment strategies may not apply to all clients, or a client may wish to consider other options.

Often clients will be curious specifically about the use of medication. The BA conceptualization of depression acknowledges that biochemical factors or familial transmission may increase vulnerability to depression and that biological changes are an essential component of the phenomenology of depression. At the same time, there are multiple ways to diminish depression and to minimize the risks of future depressive episodes. The BA conceptualization, while solidly based in the behavioral model, is chiefly a clinical tool. We often tell clients that the aim of BA is to find the exact ingredients for a "behavioral antidepressant" that will influence their mood as effectively as a "pharmaceutical antidepressant." We also describe the data supporting BA, highlighting research studies such as the Seattle study we discussed in Chapter 1, which found that BA works as well as medication and yet avoids the unfavorable side effects common to antidepressant medications. Unlike medication, BA also teaches skills that may offer more enduring protection from depression.

Other clients may be curious about the similarities and differences between BA and cognitive therapy. We generally explain to clients that the two approaches share a similar structure but that they emphasize different methods of changing depression. One of us (S. D.) once gave a detailed explanation of these differences to a client, who responded immediately, "So, are you saying that cognitive therapists believe that the head teaches the hands, whereas the BA approach assumes that the hands teach the head?" We thought this was a perfect summation of the basic differences between the two approaches, and we share it often with other clients who raise questions about cognitive therapy.

> *Principle 3:* The clues to figuring out what will be antidepressant for a particular client lie in what precedes and follows the client's important behaviors.

Clients often start treatment feeling demoralized and hopeless about the prospect of finding relief from their depression. The job of the BA therapist is to engage the client in a careful and detailed examination of what behaviors are associated with being depressed and what happens before and after such behaviors occur. It is in these examinations that the pathway out of depression may be found. Alicia's dilemma serves as a good example. After Alicia lost the job she had previously enjoyed, she began to experience disappointment with other areas of her life. Alicia had a small dog that had long been the center of attention at home. She had been in the habit of taking her dog for a walk early in the morning before work and later in the afternoon. During her time of unemployment, she took the dog to the park later in the morning and saw mostly mothers with their babies at the park where she walked. She felt lonely and out of place, and, because she was having a hard time getting up early in the morning, she stopped walking the dog altogether rather than resuming the early morning walks. She managed to go early one morning and felt a wave of anxiety as she saw people running and thought about them as gainfully employed people getting a jog in before going to work. She also felt exhausted and cranky because she had not slept well. She got testy with her dog and cut the walk short after the dog pulled at the lead one too many times. She determined not to walk that early in the morning again. She had ceased to engage in a behavior that was previously rewarding to her.

Alicia also gained about 15 pounds and felt out of shape. She would think about taking the dog for a walk and then talk herself out of going. She spent much of her time distracting herself with computer games or reading even though she knew she needed to find employment. When she had taken the lower-paying temporary job and moved into a small apartment, not only did she feel guilty about keeping her dog cooped up, but also her guilt contributed to avoiding her friends. She assumed they would judge her for taking such terrible care of her dog, and this feeling made it even more difficult to call them. She had been very vocal in the past about people needing to give their dogs plenty of exercise, and she was now doing the very thing for which she had so harshly judged others. Her depression and avoidance led to her becoming increasingly isolated, increasingly irritable, and overwhelmed most of the time. In fact, she had begun to experience intense anxiety during the wee hours of the morning that kept her awake for at least an hour with waves of nausea. She would lie in bed, fearing that the best parts of her life were over and that she would never know success again.

The life events of losing her job and moving into a small apartment had a negative impact on Alicia, as her life was less rewarding. There were a number of important clues to possible antidepressant and depressant behaviors in the patterns that followed these larger life events. Not walking her dog was antecedent to ruminating and feeling guilty, and Alicia subsequently avoided friends. The isolation was antecedent to feeling irritable and overwhelmed with worry, which kept her awake nights. She then stayed in bed later or distracted herself with computer games. Walking her dog when she was tired resulted in her being irritable with the dog, and that in turn made her feel guilty and less likely to walk the dog or even call friends. This cycle suggested that addressing the behavior of avoiding friends, passively playing computer games rather than facing the situations that made her anxious, and walking her dog all were important behaviors that could be antidepressant as she was guided through a plan for behavior change. BA therapists use activity monitoring charts to understand clients' behavior and the connections between their behaviors and moods.

Principle 4: Structure and schedule activities that follow a plan, not a mood.

Acting from the inside out works well in many situations, but it is not an effective strategy when one is depressed. For many people, the primary feeling when depressed is the feeling of not wanting to do anything at all. When we asked one BA client what he was interested in doing lately, he said clearly, "The only thing I want to do when I am depressed is *not* do!" The problem is that doing less when depressed leaves a person wanting to do even less. It can easily become a vicious cycle. Over time, not only are motivation and energy very low, but also the demands of one's life become more stressful.

BA therapists encourage people to begin acting from the "outside-in." We ask people to experiment with acting according to a goal, as opposed to acting according to a mood. Engaging in activities that once brought pleasure or a sense of accomplishment or that solve problems can improve mood and reduce life stressors over time. A core part of BA is to begin to act, even when mood and motivation are low, rather than waiting for one's mood to improve prior to getting engaged.

Throughout BA some form of activity structuring and scheduling is used to support acting from the outside-in. These strategies can be accomplished by creating detailed schedules with tasks broken down into components and assigned at specific times and places. They can also be accomplished by clearly zeroing in on one or two activities and getting a commitment from the client to engage in them at some specific time during the week. Activity structuring and scheduling is the backbone of BA, and all other strategies coalesce around these important basics.

Principle 5: Change will be easier when starting small.

Both clients and therapists can expect too much, too quickly. Change is difficult for many people, even in the best of moods, in the best of times. When one is depressed, especially if there are associated feelings of hopelessness, changing one's behavior can be a tremendous struggle. Many clients experience the prospect of change as overwhelming; others experience frustration if changes are not 100% complete. Just as cognitive therapists identify "all-or-nothing" thinking, we also see "all-or-nothing" behaving. Sometimes our clients talk about the "Nike" approach to behavior and chide themselves for their failure to "Just do it!" BA treatment depends on helping clients make changes by taking a stepwise approach. One job of an effective BA therapist is to break down any behavior into its extremely small elements, or component behaviors. Correspondingly, a potential pitfall for a therapist is failing to notice when his or her clients are taking on too much, too soon, which can be a set-up for more discouragement and despair.

Part of the art of BA, in fact, lies in finding just the right place to encourage and the right place to hold back. For instance, one client, who had been a marathon runner prior to becoming depressed, discussed his intention to exercise and his expectation that this would improve his mood. The therapist fully supported this plan. When the client began to talk about starting with 45-minute runs a few days a week, however, the therapist interjected a note of caution. Together the therapist and client worked to break down this ambitious goal into its component parts, focusing on what could get the client off to an effective start without inadvertently increasing the risk of subsequent hopelessness and discouragement. They decided that prior to the next session he would start by buying a pair of athletic shoes and shorts. In this way, tasks need to be broken down into their component parts and each part tackled successfully before moving on to the next.

Principle 6: Emphasize activities that are naturally reinforcing.

The ultimate aim of modifying behaviors in BA is to help clients engage in life in such a way as to increase the likelihood that antidepressant behaviors will be reinforced naturally by the world around them. Behaviorists often discuss differences between what they have termed "natural" reinforcement versus "arbitrary" reinforcement. In BA, the emphasis is on maximizing opportunities for the natural reinforcement of nondepressed behavior, but arbitrary reinforcers are used on occasion as well. For example, during therapy a client who has avoided social contact while depressed begins to practice reengaging coworkers in conversation. When a coworker smiles and expresses interest in the client's communication, the client continues the conversation. In this way, the client receives natural reinforcement from his or her environment. The coworker's behaviors are natural reinforcers insofar as they naturally follow the client's behavior. In contrast, giving oneself a caramel after completing an hour of housework is an arbitrary reinforcer, as such reinforcement is not naturally linked to the immediate environmental reward (in contrast to a clean house and sense of accomplishment that are possible natural rewards in such a case).

At times, however, it is also important that BA clients learn to reinforce themselves for their behavior as they attain short-term goals, given that not all behaviors are reinforced immediately and not all environments are benevolent. Often, in fact, as clients begin to activate, the environment punishes them. For instance, the client's initial attempts to engage coworkers may be met with dismissal, given the client's previously withdrawn style. In such cases, the client would need to reinforce him- or herself for taking action despite the immediate aversive consequences. Dieting is a behavior in which initial activities can be met with punishing consequences. Sometimes one experiences only minimal change after a week of careful attention to healthy eating. Someone in this situation would need to find something other than the numbers on the scale to reinforce, and thus maintain, the dieting behavior. The person could do something like putting $20 in a jar for every week on the diet to save for the purchase of a special item of clothing. Keeping up with the diet will eventually pay off in weight loss, but the dieter may need to use arbitrary self-reinforcement along the way. Similarly, a depressed client who has been unemployed for several months may experience distress upon starting to look online for job postings and to send résumés. Such a client may benefit from rewarding him- or herself by allowing equal time watching a favorite television show after spending a specified amount of time working on the job search.

Arbitrary self-reinforcement procedures have been important parts of some treatments for depression (Rehm, 1977) and are clearly used in BA as well. The emphasis of BA therapists, however, is on helping clients come into contact with the natural reinforcers in the environment. The advantage of natural rewards over arbitrary reinforcement is that natural reinforcers automatically follow the behavior and need not be concocted; so, the behavior is more likely to continue during a person's normal routine (Sulzer-Azaroff & Mayer, 1991).

Principle 7: Act as a coach.

The metaphor of a coach helps to guide the BA therapist. Good coaches help team members plan strategies, make suggestions, give direction, and keep up morale—but they don't go in and play the game for the team. The BA therapist's job is to be an effective problem solver and to encourage clients to take action to connect with rewards and to solve problems. Making changes when a person is depressed is hard, and the therapist has expertise in the principles of behavior change. Passivity is inherent in depression and can become a way of life for those who are chronically depressed. Coaching involves encouragement, as some depressed people may underestimate their ability to cope with many life problems or look at all problems as out of their control (Brown & Seigel, 1988). Coaching also involves helping to guide the process of change and make suggestions when necessary. Compassionate therapists may want to solve the problem for the client, but the good BA therapist maintains a coaching stance and allows clients to become more confident about their own game.

In addition to being an effective strategist and cheerleader for the client, part of the therapist's role as a coach is to structure therapy sessions so that the treatment stays on track. Sessions are structured to promote the most efficient use of the 45- or 50-minute hour. An agenda is set in each session during the first 5 or 10 minutes. During the early weeks of therapy the therapist may control the agenda more than the client since it is necessary to assess the client's problems, conduct a functional analysis (e.g., Yoman, 2008), and present a case conceptualization and treatment plan to the client. As an effective coach, the BA therapist also will be on the alert for ways to promote the client's active involvement even early in therapy, asking repeatedly for the client to add any important items to the agenda. In later therapy sessions the client will control the agenda, based on his or her weekly experiences. Every session should include a discussion of the previous session's homework as well as the assignment of new homework for the following session.

Principle 8: Emphasize a problem-solving empirical approach, and recognize that all results are useful.

If getting activated and engaged were easy, clients would do it themselves. A therapist cannot help a client simply by saying "Go to a movie, you'll feel better." How often have most depressed people heard that kind of statement or told themselves the same thing? BA suggests that effective therapy is an ongoing process of developing, evaluating, and trying out potential solutions. As such, it requires an ongoing problem-solving empirical approach on the part of the therapist. We encourage an experimental approach that focuses on trying a behavior and observing the outcome. In BA, the experiments are based on functional analyses of past behavior and hypotheses regarding potentially reinforcing activities for each client.

For instance, a therapist might assume that a client who was socially anxious prior to being depressed but who enjoyed working on cars is more likely to be rewarded by going to an antique car show or fixing a lawn mower than going to a party. This assumption would need to be tested, given that it is not possible to know beforehand what will reinforce a particular behavior or whether the environment will provide appropriate reinforcement for any class of behaviors. And, of course, it is preferable to test out behaviors more than once. Just as laboratory experiments need to be conducted and then replicated, so do experiments in therapy. BA therapists and clients work to plan activities on multiple occasions and try a variety of activities, evaluating the impact on clients' mood, productivity, or satisfaction with their lives prior to determining whether or not any behavior is worth continuing.

While clients in BA can become discouraged when they plan and try activities and still don't feel better, it is important for therapists to remain positive and hopeful. We learn by our successes and by our failures. When a client complains that trying an assignment didn't help, the problem-solving attitude of the BA therapist suggests a different approach. The therapist may say: "Now we know something new. We know that there is never a guarantee that changing a specific activity will help, and now we can guess that this particular activity you tried did not succeed. So, let's discuss some alternatives for the next week." The therapist would then continue a discussion about what actually happened. In some cases, a client may report he or she really tried to engage but in fact made only a half-hearted attempt. In other cases, the activity seemed potentially useful but ultimately wasn't effective in changing mood. Another possibility is that the environmental conditions in which the behavior occurred did not provide adequate reinforcement. For example, a client with a plan to talk to a friend for 20 minutes may have called the friend during a time when the friend had a head cold and was distracted. There is something to be learned from all client behaviors. The therapist's stance of remaining curious about all that can be learned from these experiences and maintaining an attitude that problem solving, rather than instant success, is key to keeping therapy moving forward both help clients to remain hopeful about making changes in their lives.

Principle 9: Don't just talk, do!

Activity is the heart of the BA approach. Thus, homework is required in each and every session. It is the crux of every treatment strategy; yet, it can be the bane of the therapist's (and client's) existence. To begin with, the word *homework* is often associated with something aversive, and so it may more usefully be referred to by another name—such as "between-session assignment" (Martell et al., 2001). Most adults are not fooled by a mere name change, though. Homework requires clients to engage in an activity between sessions. and, for depressed clients, this is often not easy to do. Above all else, homework needs to be developed *in collaboration with* the client. There are several guidelines that can help maximize success.

In setting up homework assignments with clients, the task(s) must be kept realistic. Clients also should not be expected to simply rely on willpower to engage in an agreed-upon assignment. The therapist should take time to discuss a plan of implementation with the client. The more specific and detailed the plan, the better! What will he or she need in order to be more likely to engage in the task? In the example of Alicia taking her dog for walks, she should decide on the specific times of day to take her walks and specify the length of the walks. The length and times of the walks should be reasonable, given her current schedule. She should write down the planned walk on an activity chart or in a personal calendar. She will also need to make sure that she has comfortable walking shoes available and that the dog's leash is handy at the times of the walks. Likewise, she will need to have comfortable clothing (appropriate for a variety of weather conditions) clean and on hand. Having a public commitment to another person can also increase the likelihood that an assignment will be completed. Alicia can either simply tell a friend that she plans to walk on a particular morning and commit to calling the friend when the walk is completed, or she can make a date to walk with a friend, increasing the obligation and, ultimately, the potential for actually engaging in the task.

A fundamental error that therapists make when assigning activities between sessions is to neglect to review them in the following session. Homework compliance may be extinguished if it is not rewarded. If it is assigned, it needs to be reviewed. When a client reports failure to complete an assignment, the therapist and client need to conduct an analysis of the problems that resulted in the task not being completed. If the report is that the client was successful, this provides a great opportunity to discuss increasing the frequency or intensity of the activity during the next week.

Principle 10: Troubleshoot possible and actual barriers to activation.

Although it would be a wonderful achievement for us to say that we had discovered the way to motivate all clients, guarantee that they will complete therapy homework, and keep them fully engaged in treatment, we have not yet discovered such a magic formula for each and every client. BA, like all other therapies, requires persistence and creativity on the part of the therapist and the client. It is a basic principle of BA that problems will arise and that troubleshooting possible and actual barriers to activation is essential. Therapists promote activation by anticipating barriers to client's completing activity assignments or monitoring tasks and by troubleshooting when a difficulty has occurred in order to reduce the likelihood that same problem will continue in the future.

Summary

The 10 principles enumerated in Table 2.1 describe the basic guidelines to BA therapy. BA therapists firmly subscribe to the principle that changing what clients do will have a positive impact on their feelings (Principle 1). Therapists present clients with an initial case conceptualization and seek their buy-in for the treatment, using the framework that changes in life can lead to depression and that there are natural reactions to life changes that result in coping efforts that keep people stuck (Principle 2). By monitoring the client's behavior and mood connections closely, therapists focus in on keys to behavior change by noticing what precedes and follows important behaviors (Principle 3), structuring and scheduling relevant activities (Principle 4), making small changes and building on those (Principle 5), and targeting behaviors that are likely to be naturally rewarded in the client's environment (Principle 6). BA therapists act as a coach who helps to plan the steps that clients will ultimately be responsible for playing out (Principle 7), and the overarching goal is for clients to become their own coach. As BA is a solution-focused therapy, the therapist takes a problem-solving stance. Both therapist and client collaborate in an experimental approach to trying new behaviors and discovering important results of behavior change (Principle 8). BA is an active therapy. What happens between sessions is of greater importance in many ways than the actual therapy hour itself. BA is not about talking about problems—it is about doing activities that can lead to improvements in life situations or moods (Principle 9). Finally, BA therapists and clients continue to work together to identify possible barriers to activation or actual problems that have occurred and to troubleshoot methods for resolving difficulties (Principle 10).

Putting the Principles into Practice

This book is intended as one that you keep readily available on your desk, occasionally consulting it before sessions to plan interventions. The following chapters will help you to identify treatment targets and conduct a functional analysis as part of assessment and treatment, thereby providing concrete applications for Principles 1–3. Throughout the book, we will refer to examples from Alicia's story as well as brief examples from others. The story of Alicia is not intended to represent a session-by-session protocol, and examples are used to illustrate various interventions rather than to describe what therapy looks like from beginning to end. Examples of therapy from start to finish can be found elsewhere (Martell et al., 2001; Dimidjian, Martell, Addis, & Herman-Dunn, 2008). We devote a fair amount of attention to activation strategies such as activity monitoring and activity scheduling, which are the foci of Principles 3, 4, 5, 6, and 9. We present how to take a problem-solving stance and troubleshoot when the treatment does not seem to be going as planned, which follows the overarching Principles 7, 8, and 10. Because avoidance behavior is so prevalent in depression and breaking patterns of avoidance so essential to BA, avoidance modification strategies will be considered repeatedly. When BA was developed, it was done in the context of a clinical trial comparing the behavioral aspects of cognitive therapy to the full cognitive therapy protocol. Thus, when therapists in the study needed to confront clients who were stuck in negative thinking, they needed to do so from a behavioral rather than a cognitive perspective. In BA, thinking is considered a problematic behavior, and the act of ruminating over one's distress is a target of the intervention. We devote an entire chapter (Chapter 7) to this important topic. Finally, we discuss future directions for BA as a treatment as well as for the clients you work with as we wrap up with unanswered questions for the profession and also discuss relapse prevention techniques for clients.

3

The Structure
and Style of Therapy

I think one's feelings waste themselves in words, they ought all
to be distilled into actions and into actions which bring results.
—FLORENCE NIGHTINGALE (1820–1919)

Alicia felt apprehensive about her second session as she walked
into Beth's office building. She had read over the booklet[1] on BA that
Beth had given her at the end of their first session. She felt a combination of curiosity and discouragement. She was interested in learning
more about the approach to depression that was described. At the
same time, she felt demoralized. She just wasn't sure it was for her. "It
all makes sense," she thought, "but I just can't imagine how it's going
to make any difference for me." As soon as she had the thought, she
felt worse, thinking, "This is so typical of me, I'm not even in the
door and I'm already giving up. It's pathetic."

Beth seemed happy to see Alicia as she entered the office. She
greeted her warmly and asked if Alicia would be willing to fill out
the same questionnaire about depression that she filled out before
the last session. As they sat down, Beth explained that she would
ask Alicia to fill out the same questionnaire each time they met in
order to learn about how Alicia was doing and to assess the degree to
which the therapy was working. Beth commented: "From what you

---

[1]The booklet referred to here is "Beginning Activation Therapy for Depression: A
Self-Help Manual," which can be found in Martell, Addis, and Jacobson (2001, pp.
202–205).

are answering this week, it looks like you are feeling about the same as last week, although it looks like your sleep is a little worse. Does that seem accurate to you?" Alicia was surprised that Beth seemed genuinely interested in the fine details of how she was doing. She reflected on the last 2 weeks: "Yes, that is about right. Things are just pretty bad overall, and I am spending a lot of time in bed, but I don't know if I ever really get restful sleep. I'm so miserable and worry all the time that I'll be broke and have nobody in my life."

As Beth was making some notes on the questionnaire, Alicia realized that she wasn't sure what to expect from therapy or what she was supposed to say or do now that she was here. She felt relieved when Beth began to explain, "Alicia, I was hoping we could start by talking a little bit about how this therapy works." "That sounds good," said Alicia and continued with some hesitation, "It's not personal, but I never really wanted to see a therapist. I have no idea how this is supposed to go." Beth didn't seem bothered at all by what she had said; in fact, her voice was kind as she replied, "That makes total sense to me, Alicia. It's often really difficult to start therapy for the first time. It wouldn't surprise me if you had a million questions but weren't sure how to even begin with one of them." That's exactly how I feel, thought Alicia, as she nodded quietly.

"I know the booklet talked a little about this, but I think it's really important as we get started to emphasize that this therapy is both collaborative and structured. This means that each time we meet we'll begin by making a plan together for our session. I call this our 'agenda' for the session. The reason for making an agenda together is that it can help us stay on track with addressing the topics that are most important to you. Does this sound okay?" Alicia thought that made good sense to her. "From my standpoint, there are two areas I was hoping we could address today," said Beth, "First, I wanted to talk some more about the general approach of BA and how it might fit for you. And, second, I was hoping we could talk about how we can best work together."

When Beth had finished explaining her goals for the session, she added, "Do you have anything else you want to make sure we address today?" Alicia was surprised again; Beth really seemed invested in involving her. "I was wondering if we could talk about what it said in the booklet about activity making you less tired. It didn't make a lot of sense. I'm so tired all the time. It's not really realistic to be active when you are this exhausted." "Absolutely!" said Beth. "I'm going to write that down for our agenda, and we'll make sure to address that today. That's a great topic to add."

Introduction

Like Alicia, when clients first come to therapy, they are frequently unsure what to expect. Many are unfamiliar with BA, and, in fact, few start therapy wanting to activate themselves more. It is the very nature of depression to pull away and decrease activity. As Alicia expressed, it is hard to imagine how to get active when feeling exhausted all the time. Many depressed clients come to therapy believing that they need to feel better before they can get active and make changes in their lives. How can this therapy work if one needs to feel motivated before taking action? As Alicia's therapist illustrated, it is important to begin therapy by responding directly to these types of questions and concerns.

BA is a structured treatment, and during early sessions it is important to explain some of the key elements of the structure. In this chapter, we will review these key elements, including the BA model of depression and change that sets the context for the overall course of treatment. We also will address how to explain the roles of the therapist and client and the importance of homework. Finally, we will discuss the structure of each BA session, including the importance of reviewing progress since the last contact, setting an agenda, orienting to new procedures used, and maintaining a focus on activation throughout the session. Near the end of therapy the structure of the sessions includes a focus on consolidating gains and planning for relapse prevention. After a course of BA the therapist and client will be able to anticipate triggers for behaviors that increase depressive symptoms and develop a plan for alternative activities that can help the client to cope in these situations.

BA is also characterized by a number of key structural and stylistic strategies. For instance, in her second session with Alicia, Beth expressed genuine warmth and interest in Alicia's experience. When Alicia expressed reluctance to start therapy, Beth responded in a matter-of-fact and nonjudgmental manner. She reinforced Alicia's sharing of her questions and concerns with encouragement, and she invited Alicia to be an active participant in therapy. In this chapter, we review these stylistic qualities, which are essential elements of doing BA.

The Structure of BA: Activation Is the Guide

The basic structure of BA is guided, most fundamentally, by a focus on activation. The first and second principles of BA define this focus. The first principle of BA summarizes the model of change: "*The key to changing how people feel is to help them change what they do.*" This principle communicates the premise that when clients wait to feel motivated they remain in the endless cycle. Given this dilemma, we ask them to work from the "outside-in" as opposed to the "inside-out" (Martell et al., 2001). In other words, the structure of BA is focused on committing to action regardless of how clients feel inside and anticipating that motivation will follow, rather than the other way around. As therapists, we work as coaches to help with this very challenging method of working from the "outside-in." We help to break down activities to increase the likelihood that the client, even with extremely low motivation, will do them. We also help clients to develop structure in their daily lives in order to increase the likelihood of acting according to their goals.

The second principle of BA summarizes the model of depression, which defines the focus on activation in BA: "*Changes in life can lead to depression, and short-term coping strategies may keep people stuck over time.*" This principle establishes the structure for knowing what to assess and target in therapy. There are many theories of depression, all of which likely speak to aspects of this heterogeneous disorder. The model of depression that guides BA is consistent with behavioral models articulated decades ago (e.g., Lewinsohn, 1974).

The early models of depression highlighted that when people's lives are low in positive reinforcement or high in punishment, depression is more likely. How does this happen? Under such conditions, people may learn that their actions do not result in anything desirable, or they may learn instead to focus on how to escape or avoid a punishing environment. In effect, people learn to pull back from life and stop engaging. Although pulling back from life in this way is natural and understandable, it can also keep one stuck in depression. The less one does, the less one wants to do; and the less one does, the more likely it is that problems in one's life will build and accumulate. As access to positive reinforcement is decreased and experience of punishment is increased, a vicious cycle of depression can develop. There is a heightened state of self-awareness as the individual attempts to reduce the impact of these disruptions and is unable to do so. Increases in self-consciousness and dysphoria lead to the cognitive, behavioral, and emotional changes that are correlated with depression and reduce the individual's ability to cope with future depression-evoking events. Components of this downward spiral have been described by Lewinsohn and colleagues (Lewinsohn, 1974; Lewinsohn & Graf, 1973) as well as others (e.g., Beck et al., 1979).

It makes sense that individuals try to reduce the impact of emotional disruptions. However, the behaviors in which they engage, such as negative ruminations on distress, escape from or avoidance of aversive experiences, and attempts to avoid emotional pain, serve to reduce contact with potential reinforcers in the environment. This withdrawal keeps the depressed individual stuck in a pattern of feeling bad. Eventually emotions are shut down, and the individual feels worse and increasingly more depressed and hopeless about the prospect of change. The chief tasks for the BA therapist and client are to identify contingencies (i.e., the situations in which the behavior occurs and the consequences of the behavior) that make action more likely and to define treatment targets that will result in the client's building a better life, thereby reducing depressive symptoms.

We often find it helpful to use a visual depiction of the BA model of depression. Such diagrams can aid therapists in developing a comprehensive case conceptualization. In addition, such diagrams are often useful in explaining the basic model to clients. It is important in using such diagrams (and in explaining the model generally) to be sensitive to the fact that every person has a unique life history. Although the principles of BA apply generally, every client has a unique case formulation in BA. Helping clients to understand how the events in their lives influence the experience and impacts of depression can be very validating and is a key part of starting treatment in BA.

Figure 3.1 provides a diagram that may be used to develop a case conceptualization and to explain the BA model of depression to their clients. The first question that we ask is "What happened in the client's context that triggered or made likely the conditions for depression?" The third principle, that "*The clues to figuring out*

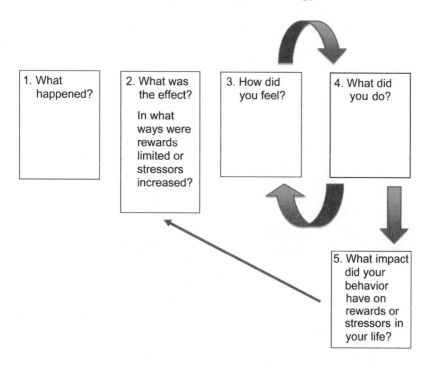

FIGURE 3.1. The BA model of depression.

what will be antidepressant for a particular client lie in what precedes and what follows the client's important behaviors," is key to understanding the kinds of behaviors that have been reinforced in the past and those that were not reinforced or were punished. Often, clients will report events that occurred in their lives, such as losses of relationships or jobs, financial losses or burdens, and changes such as the birth of a child, caring for aging relatives, and even ongoing daily hassles. At times, clients will highlight biological factors, and we explain that both biological and environmental factors come into play in understanding life events. Although it's not the way we commonly think about "life events," in BA the notion of events can be expanded to encompass both external and internal experience. We then examine the impact of these events, focusing in particularly on the ways in which access to rewards is limited or stressors are increased over time. Then, we turn to the effects of living in this sort of context on how the client feels. Often, depressed clients will say,

TABLE 3.1. Frequently Asked Questions and Sample Answers

- *Isn't depression caused by a chemical imbalance in my brain?*
  Answer: We know that our biology is related to depression, and we also know that changing our behavior can impact our body's chemistry. Depression is a complex condition that has multiple causes. Fortunately, depression is also a very treatable problem, and many different types of treatment have been shown to help.

- *What about medications?*
  Answer: Antidepressant medications are effective for many people. The type of psychotherapy that I offer, behavioral activation, also has been demonstrated to be an effective treatment for depression. In addition, research suggests that the effects of BA can last after the treatment is completed; this tells us that the benefits of what people learn in BA can help them prevent getting depressed again in the future, even after they finish therapy.

- *Isn't this approach too simple?*
  Answer: The ideas in this approach are straightforward, but putting them into practice can be difficult. That is why my role is to be a coach for you in the process of change. As we work together, I can help to guide you through a process of taking steps to get active, solve problems in your life, and feel better. It is a powerful approach, but I often say that if this were so simple you would have done it already.

- *This "activation" business seems impossible. I can barely get out of bed. Can this really help me?*
  Answer: When you're depressed it is understandable that this would seem impossible and that you would question whether anything can work. A lot of people ask that very question, and many people find that what seems impossible at first begins to get easier as they get more active and reengaged. This approach is very practical, and my job is to help figure out how to make it manageable, how to find places and ways to begin activating that are doable for you right now. For some people, it's also helpful to remember that this approach has worked for many depressed people. All that said, I wouldn't be honest if I told you that I could guarantee success. I am committed to working together with you, starting where you are right now and building from there. My guess is that, as we move forward, this will all seem more feasible to you. If you are willing, we can start with a few small steps and observe the outcome and then move on from there.

- *Isn't it faking to act like I'm not depressed when I am?*
  Answer: People often ask this question. It may feel awkward, but it is not fake or insincere to choose to behave in a more engaged way even when you are feeling "down." By acting as if you are not depressed, you can engage in the very behaviors that can help you feel better and build a life that supports your mood and well-being.

(continued)

TABLE 3.1. (*continued*)

- *How can I add more activities when I'm already too busy and that is why I'm so depressed?*
  Answer: It may be that there are, in fact, too many things on your plate. We will take a look at how all these activities serve you. I want to help you to problem-solve getting more done, fully engaging in activities, and not feeling overwhelmed.

- *Can BA work when other treatments have not?*
  Answer: BA is not a cure-all by any means. I know from research that this approach can help individuals when they are depressed. I often ask my clients, What if we treated this like an experiment? We can work together for a period of time and see if this approach works for you. Since I can't guarantee success, shall we decide on a time when we'll discuss how things are going, say after four or five sessions? We'll be talking during that time as well about what might be working and what might not be working for you. What do you think?

Note. This table provides examples of a few questions frequently asked of BA therapists. The answers are not intended to be exhaustive responses but rather capture the essence of a typical response from the BA therapist.

"It feels awful. I feel sad, lonely, discouraged, and hopeless." One of the key elements to communicate in explaining this model is that depression is not the fault of the individual and that feeling depressed makes sense, given one's context.

Figure 3.1 also represents the vicious cycle of depression as the client engages in coping strategies to deal with depressed mood that unfortunately function to worsen the negative feelings and, over time, add to the weight of the factors that make depression more likely. For instance Alicia felt depressed following the loss of her job, and she stopped engaging in other activities. When she began to gain weight and felt like she was neglecting her dog, she spent even more time staying at home and felt increasingly out of place with her other friends. She then felt even more depressed and began to isolate herself further. A reproducible version of Figure 3.1 with space for comments is provided in Appendix 1a for use by clients in consulting their therapists.

Clients may have particular questions about BA. Table 3.1 provides a short list of frequently asked questions and example answers. Sometimes a client may object to certain features of the BA model. When therapists present the BA model of depression to clients, there may be objections to a model that underemphasizes the role of biology in depression. As we noted above, we fold biological or family predispositions to depression into our discussion of life events, like all other identifiable life events. One frequent objection to the BA model takes the form of the question "I thought depression was caused by a chemical imbalance—don't I need medication to overcome depression?" The answer to this question is multifaceted. Antidepressant medication is a viable option for many. Nevertheless, the belief that medicine works on the biological aspect while BA works on the behavioral is an arbitrary distinction. The reality is that there are biological components to all human behavior (Linehan, 2006), and changing our actions or reactions changes our biology, just as changing biochemical levels through medication may change emotional reactions and, in some cases, actions.

One other objection that warrants a brief mention here is that the model sounds too simplistic. We typically respond to this comment by acknowledging that, while the model is relatively simple and straightforward, it also integrates a well-founded understanding that overcoming depression is often very difficult. In fact, we highlight the perception that clients sometimes believe that they are being asked to do the near-impossible, namely, to get active. To address concerns about oversimplifying the process of change, we emphasize that change is usually not easy, and a critical job of the therapist is to serve as a guide or coach, as discussed earlier.

When able to do so skillfully, therapists can build the foundation of the therapeutic relationship by explaining the BA model to their depressed clients. When the model is brought to life by including details provided during the initial interview, conceptualizing the case in session affirms that the therapist has "got it" and has a beginning understanding of the client's situation. The conceptualization is always presented as a hypothesis. It would be foolish for any therapist to presume that he or she knows what caused or maintains a person's depression. However, we must make hypotheses, test them out, and provide a model that scaffolds the various strategies used in BA. There may be broad treatment goals developed initially in therapy, and clients will then develop various weekly goals. Functional analysis—that is, looking at the situations in which behavior occurs and the consequences of the behavior—is used throughout. Specifically, in order to form hypotheses about behaviors that may maintain depression, the therapist looks at the function of behaviors and how they serve a client. For example, wearing old sweatpants to run to the store may serve the function of providing comfort and allowing a person to quickly complete the errand, or it may serve the function of allowing the person to avoid the time and attention to oneself required to put together a more stylish outfit.

The Structure of Each Session

There is a general structure to all of the therapy sessions in BA. The primary structuring elements include reviewing progress since the last contact, setting an agenda, attending to the client's understanding, soliciting feedback, and using homework. In addition, the therapist structures each session by maintaining a focus on activation. These elements may vary in duration from session to session, client to client, or therapist to therapist. They may also vary in the detail allotted to each element in any given session. Despite such flexibility, however, the use of structuring strategies in each session ensures that both therapist and client remain on track in helping the client activate and engage in life.

One of the first activities that Beth asked Alicia to undertake at the start of their second (and every subsequent) session was to complete a Beck Depression Inventory–II (BDI-II; Beck & Steer, 1987), since her depression was the primary focus of treatment. In so doing, she was following one of the key structuring strategies in BA; namely, *reviewing progress since the last contact.* Many therapists working with depressed clients use a self-report scale such as the BDI-II to monitor progress during treatment. Others may ask clients to report verbally on depressed mood or other key symptoms on a 1–10 scale at the outset of each session. Such practices enable the therapist to quantify progress or the lack thereof. Clinicians may also use measures to assess comorbid disorders such as anxiety self-report scales—for example, the Beck Anxiety Inventory (Beck, Epstein, Brown, & Steer, 1988) or others. Using other formal measures is a way of monitoring additional treatment targets along with monitoring a client's mood and depression. Several collections of quantitative measures for depression (e.g., Nezu, Ronan, Meadows, & McClure, 2000) and for anxiety (e.g., Antony, Orsillo, & Roemer, 2001) provide information about empirically based measures as well as reproducible forms that can be used to implement many measures. These allow for multiple samples that may assist in better understanding the details of the client's improvement. However, therapists must balance their need for more information against the burden that too many measures may place on the client. Over time, graphing the scores from self-report measures can be helpful to both the therapist and client. Graphing scores over time can show the therapist and client when fluctuations in mood occur and can help alert the therapist as to whether treatment is working or not. When clients are steadily improving, graphing objective scores provides a hopeful visual representation of the client's gains. And when clients are not improving, conversely, monitoring progress at each session highlights the need for reviewing the assessment, case conceptualization, and/or activation plans.

Using objective measures in each session does not diminish the need for therapists to also check on other areas of progress in the client's life since the preceding session. The therapist may ask the client to provide an overall rating of mood during the preceding week or time period and also inquire about details regarding activity level. Some of this information will be provided by reviewing homework (see below), but a check-in regimen at the beginning of every session is useful for a number of reasons. It shows the client that the therapist is interested in his or her life outside the therapy hour. It also helps to set an agenda for the session when either marked improvements or deteriorations are noted.

Once the BA therapist has reviewed progress since the last contact, setting an agenda is typically the first order of business. Agenda setting is usually brief but is best when the agenda is fairly detailed, including setting priorities and how much time to spend on each item. What is most important about setting agendas is to ensure that the client is encouraged to suggest topics of importance to him or her and that the therapist has kept in mind topics that maintain a focus on activation in order to help the client achieve his or her goals. Thus, like most cognitive and behavioral therapies, agenda setting is a collaborative process that involves encouraging the client to contribute items for the agenda, setting priorities, and negotiating changes that may occur as the session unwinds. If the session subsequently veers away from the agreed-upon agenda, the therapist should check in with the client to ensure that that course is acceptable and that both the therapist and client agree that the detour is in the service of the client's goals and priorities.

Another key element of the way in which the BA therapist structures each session involves the use of orienting as well as soliciting feedback. *Orienting* helps to "take the mystery out of therapy," as our friend and colleague Marsha Linehan says, and gives clients the rationale for the procedures to be used. *Soliciting feedback* helps to ensure that clients understand such procedures. We have already discussed orienting to the BA model, which is typically done during the first or second sessions of therapy (however, the therapist may, and frequently does, return to the model over the course of treatment). During each session, the therapist also orients the client to the procedures used. For example, we ask clients to monitor activity for a specific reason. Such monitoring helps the client and therapist gather information about behavior patterns and activity/mood connections. It is important in BA to explain such rationales to the client prior to assigning an activity chart. It is also important to solicit feedback about the degree to which clients have understood and agree with such rationales.

Each session of BA is also structured to make heavy use of *homework*. Thus, in each session, the BA therapist will review the homework assigned in the preceding session and assign new tasks for the client to engage in prior to the next session. The cardinal rule of any behavioral or cognitive-behavioral therapy is that any homework assigned must be reviewed during the following session. Homework helps to reengage the client in life and reinforces the experience of BA as an action-oriented treatment. Various types of homework assignments include:

- *Activity and mood monitoring.* This will be discussed in further detail in Chapter 4, as it is an essential part of BA. Monitoring assignments are standard assignments in early sessions and may be used in later sessions in modified form.

- *Activity scheduling.* This type of homework is discussed in detail in Chapter 5, and constitutes the bulk of work completed in BA.

- *Activity structuring/grading tasks.* It is often helpful to break big tasks in life into manageable parts, and this is especially true for people with depression. During depressive episodes, tasks that appear simple can be extremely difficult. Therefore, it takes a great amount of skill to break down seemingly small tasks into even smaller units. We discuss grading tasks in more detail in Chapter 5.

- *Attention-to-experience exercises.* These types of activities are assigned when clients spend a great deal of time ruminating. Rumination is a private behavior that often interferes with full engagement in activities. We discuss attention-to-experience exercises in more detail in Chapter 7.

- *Maintaining an activation focus.* The final element of structuring that an effective BA therapist uses is *maintaining an activation focus* throughout each session. Keeping sessions focused on activation means bringing all discussions back to what the client may *do* that will improve his or her life situation or mood. Thus, the therapist frequently will redirect the conversation to the here and now and to a discussion of a potential action plan, keeping in the forefront of his or her mind the question, What can the client *do?*

Maintaining an activation focus need not be done in such a fashion as to suggest that the therapist is not interested in the client's inner life or problematic past. As we discuss in more detail in Chapter 4, it is possible to maintain an activation focus even when conducting assessment and discussing past experiences of the client. When a BA therapist talks with clients about their past, he or she does so in the context of the case formulation. This information provides hypotheses about reinforcement and punishment contingencies in the client's life. This information is used as a guide to what clients can do in the here and now and potential ways in which they can reengage. For example, Alicia had been very hurt long ago when her mother kicked her out of their house. Although she eventually reestablished a cordial relationship with her mother, she remained disengaged from her two younger siblings. In therapy, she talked about how sad she felt about the incident with her mother and the acute pain that she still felt. It was difficult for her even to talk about this with Beth. When the conversation turned to feelings of sadness, anger, guilt, or shame about this situation, Beth structured the conversation to address ways that Alicia could approach such feelings rather than avoid them and activate in the direction of important goals. By talking about the difficult feelings and allowing herself to feel them in therapy, she also created an opportunity to think of ways that she could slowly reestablish relationships with her younger siblings, something that she strongly desired but was equally afraid of.

ALICIA: I can't stop thinking about the last year when things with my mother were at the worst. She said so many terrible things about me in front of my sister and brother. Sometimes I think they were true, and it makes me feel so badly about myself. I think that my brother and sister also think these things are true. I've never been able to talk with them about how difficult Mom was when I was young. She was drinking a lot then, and I got pretty rebellious. By the time they were old enough to pay attention, Mom had stopped drinking, but her relationship with me was terrible. I think they blame me.

BETH: It seems like you feel really stuck wanting to connect with your sister and brother but that it also makes you feel really bad when you think about doing so. Did you spend a great deal of time over the past week thinking about this?

ALICIA: It was mostly on Sunday. I thought I'd call my sister to just say "hello." It was Sunday, though, and that is always the pits. We also spent many Sundays just pretending to be happy while my Mom was well on her way to being drunk. I'd just get really mad and blow up about what a bunch of crap that was. My sister remembers some of my blow-ups. It's like I ruined her Sundays, but she just doesn't know how awful it was for me.

BETH: So, you were thinking about this on Sunday, and you then decided not to call her?

ALICIA: Yes. I actually think about it a lot. Especially the fights my mother and I had in front of them. She blamed me for most of our problems. I wonder whether my sister and brother blame me as well.

BETH: So, you don't want to have that brought up when you call. Was there anything you were looking forward to talking about with your sister?

ALICIA: I know she has a new cat, and I'd love to hear about it. She may also have some thoughts about my work situation. She's really smart and usually helpful when I do call her. I just don't call very much, and I think she'd be shocked and I'd feel like I had to make excuses for not calling sooner.

BETH: So, you avoided feeling bad and experiencing the crummy Sunday reminders, but you also missed the benefits that you sometimes get from talking to her.

ALICIA: I had even thought that I might suggest we do a video call over the computer so she could show me her cat. I think it is a kitten. I thought it might be fun to see if my dog would see it and go nuts. But I just don't want to be reminded of how much better my mom was to her than to me, or how much she blames me for all the stuff we lived through. That would make me feel even more alone, like I was just the jerk who ruined everyone's life back then.

BETH: Alicia, it makes total sense that you wouldn't want to feel that way or think those thoughts about yourself. Still, what you are telling me is that you also want to get the benefits of talking to her. Are there other days that could work for calling her that wouldn't be quite as bad as Sunday?

ALICIA: Yes.

BETH: Are there any days when you think you'd be more likely to enjoy calling her?

ALICIA: I guess it would be easier to call on a Friday evening. She'd be done with her workweek, and it doesn't feel so much like the awful Sundays.

BETH: Then you think you'd have an easier time if you were to call her on a different day?

ALICIA: I suppose.

BETH: Do you want to talk about ways to plan that in for this coming week?

Beth worked with Alicia to focus on what concrete steps she could take in the present to address the important goal of developing a closer relationship with her younger sister. In the process, Beth and Alicia examined relevant aspects of Alicia's history; however, the focus of the conversation returned directly to what Alicia could do differently to activate in the direction of this important life goal.

In summary, structuring sessions in BA is consistent with other behavioral and cognitive-behavioral therapies in that the treatment is goal-directed and each session follows an agenda set collaboratively by the client and therapist. There is not a specific session-by-session structure to BA, and the treatment may look quite different from client to client. The guiding principles provide structure to the therapist, who adjusts his or her style to a particular client and helps activate

TABLE 3.2. Style and Stance of an Effective BA Therapist

- Maintain session structure.
- Remain action-oriented.
- Validate clients' experiences.
- Work collaboratively with clients.
- Be nonjudgmental.
- Express warmth and be genuine with clients.
- Reinforce reports or examples of adaptive behavior.

From *Behavioral Activation for Depression: A Clinician's Guide* by Christopher R. Martell, Sona Dimidjian, and Ruth Herman-Dunn. Copyright 2010 by The Guilford Press. Permission to photocopy this table is granted to purchasers of this book for personal use only (see copyright page for details). Purchasers may download a larger version of this table from the book's page on The Guilford Press website.

clients to increase the likelihood that they will contact positive reinforcers and increasingly engage in antidepressant behavior.

Style of the Therapist

BA is an action-oriented treatment, and the style with which the therapist structures treatment and promotes activity is critical. In this section, we discuss some of the key aspects of a therapist's style (summarized in Table 3.2) including validation, collaboration, a nonjudgmental stance, being warm and genuine, and working to reinforce reports of or examples of adaptive behavior in session. Many of these stylistic strategies are consistent with other psychotherapies and do not necessarily represent unique elements of BA. This overlap, however, makes them no less important in BA. The ways in which a therapist interacts with a client about the process of change play an essential role in the BA approach.

Validation

Validating a client means demonstrating an understanding of the client's experience. Validation has been written about extensively in behavioral therapy literature (e.g., Linehan, 1993) and plays a significant role in BA. It requires all of the basic listening skills that have been widely discussed in writings on clinical practice. Being skilled at "reading" clients is a core ingredient of BA. BA therapists may use the skills of rephrasing or reflecting what clients have said.

Often, responding accurately to subtle or nonverbal communications of clients is a critical part of validation. For example, during a conversation about a social activity in which Alicia had participated, she shifted her gaze from Beth to her feet. After this continued for a couple of minutes, Beth asked, "I notice that you aren't looking at me when we talk about your dinner with Meg—has something just changed for you as we talk?" Alicia began to cry and said: "Well, I actually had a terrible time with Meg, even though we went to dinner and I said it gave me a sense of accomplishment. I felt so jealous of some of the good things that have happened to her, and I feel like a jerk for feeling that way." Had Beth not been attentive to the subtle change in the client's demeanor, she might have simply discussed the activity as one that brought a sense of accomplishment to Alicia but not as one that also generated feelings of jealousy and guilt.

Effective validation also typically involves communicating that you understand the client's experience, based on their history or current context. During the initial interviews the therapist listens carefully to the client's story about historical events that have had an impact on his or her life. The therapist reflects back to the client the life events that may have contributed to the client's depression during the presentation of the model. This is a good time to check in with the client that the therapist has fully understood the story. The therapist also uses the client's own words to talk about the symptoms of depression that the client experiences. Finally, the therapist lists the responses to the symptoms that are understandable, given the client's life history and current mood, but that may exacerbate depression, reduce access to positive reinforcement, or further complicate the client's life. Such responses to depressive symptoms can be regarded as secondary problems (Jacobson et al., 2001; Martell et al., 2001). Most clients find this process of discussing the model with the therapist to be validating and accurate in terms of their experience. If a client does not agree, the therapist needs to be open to understanding the client's perceptions of his or her experience and make modifications to the presentation of the model accordingly. To lack validation is to "miss the point" in one's interactions with one's clients, and the BA therapist works to prevent such lapses in understanding.

Appropriate validation is exemplified in this interaction between a therapist and her 78-year-old depressed client:

CLIENT: I had a really hard time getting to the post office this week to buy the stamps I needed to send the letters for last week's therapy homework.

THERAPIST: What caused the difficulty?

CLIENT: Primarily my hips and knees have really been hurting, and I just kept waiting until it would feel better to walk the six blocks I need to in order to get there. Plus I have to go up and down the flight of stairs from my apartment. I haven't needed groceries, so I just didn't go out.

THERAPIST: That makes sense to me. I'm sorry it was so painful for you. It sounds like the physical pain was a real barrier to carrying out the plan we talked about last week.

CLIENT: Yes, it was.

THERAPIST: Last week, we talked about how important it is for you to feel connected with your children, and it seemed like the plan for mailing letters to them regularly was a good one for that. I know the pain was a barrier this past week. I'm wondering, are you still thinking it is a worthwhile plan to pursue?

CLIENT: I really do. It's just that I'm not sure whether I can do it.

THERAPIST: That is a great question. Perhaps there is another way for you to get the stamps you need. Is that something we might want to talk about a little bit further today?

CLIENT: I guess so. I think you can buy stamps online these days, but I've never done that.

THERAPIST: Do you have access to get online?

CLIENT: Yes, I don't use the computer very often, but I can if I need to.

THERAPIST: Well, let's talk about some ways that you might be able to get the stamps that don't require going up and down stairs or walking around when you are in pain.

In the interaction, the therapist validated the client's difficulty in the context of his current experience. This communicated that the therapist both understood what the client was saying and viewed it as a credible and valid experience. At the same time, the therapist continued to encourage the client to move ahead on the activation plan that they discussed previously. In this way, the therapist validated the client's perspective and helped to problem-solve alternatives so that the client could still make contact with his children through letters, which was a highly desirable behavior to this client.

Collaboration

The importance of collaboration in BA permeates the treatment. Everything the therapist does in BA, from presenting the model to monitoring the client's behavior and developing activation strategies, is done in a collaborative manner with the client. Collaborative BA therapists encourage their clients to take an active role during sessions and share responsibility with them to allow them to function together as a "team." For instance, in each session therapists begin by collaboratively enlisting the client's input in setting the session agenda and end the session by collaboratively agreeing on appropriate homework.

The antithesis to collaboration in BA involves the therapist's monopolizing the session, forcing an agenda, or, at the other extreme, being excessively passive in response to the client. The therapist is the expert on activation treatment, while the client is the expert on his or her own experience. A noncollaborative therapist doesn't allow for this stance. Therapists who are unable to assume a collaborative attitude may also fail to be open to the client's influence at important junctures during the session. In contrast, collaborative therapists are responsive to client behavior and modify agendas and interventions as appropriate.

Nonjudgmental Stance

Working with depressed clients can be challenging, particularly when clients do not engage in planned behaviors or report little change in mood. For instance, a client comes in for the sixth session after having committed previously to take a shower each day. The therapist and client had worked with effort during the preceding session to design this plan carefully and specifically and ended the session feeling encouraged that they had developed a workable action plan. In this session, however, the client tells the therapist that he had a rough week and hasn't showered or left the house since the last session. At these times, it can be easy to fall into blaming clients for lack of progress or expressing frustration with them for not making changes more quickly or easily. In BA, such situations instead ask the therapist to respond in a nonjudgmental and matter-of-fact manner, neither over-reacting to nor minimizing the client's behavior. A nonjudgmental stance reduces the possibility of being perceived as treating clients in a hostile, demeaning, or critical way. Instead, the therapist maintains a focus on understanding the barriers to change and working collabora-tively with the client to develop more effective action plans. In Chapter 8, we focus in particular on how the therapist can use troubleshooting to respond nonjudgmentally to challenges to activation.

Warmth and Genuineness

A key part of doing BA is expressing warmth toward one's clients in a genuine fashion. Most therapists find it easy to experience a sense of warmth and genuine concern in relationship to their clients. The emphasis on being genuine helps to remind therapists that they can communicate such feelings in ways that are consistent with their general styles; they can simply be themselves with clients. On the other hand, therapists who do not connect with their clients on an empathic level can appear cold and uncaring. Consider an interaction in which a client tells a therapist about a very difficult loss. In the first instance, the therapist is not empathic; in the second, the therapist uses a forced and phony empathic response; and in the third example, the therapist is warm and genuine.

Example 1

CLIENT: Well, just about 5 months ago, my best friend was killed in a car accident on her way to work. I basically figured out it was her by recognizing her car on the news because I was at home sick that day.

THERAPIST: That was pretty serendipitous that you'd have seen it on television.

CLIENT: I guess. It was devastating. I called my friend's cell phone immediately, and a police officer answered and told me there had been an accident and asked if I knew how to contact her family.

THERAPIST: Uh-huh.

CLIENT: I just keep thinking about her last minutes. How scared she must have been.

THERAPIST: It seems that you are torturing yourself with these repeated thoughts. In BA we'll work on how to find some alternatives to ruminating about things that make you so upset.

Example 2

CLIENT: Well, just about 5 months ago, my best friend was killed in a car accident on her way to work. I basically figured out it was her by recognizing her car on the news because I was at home sick that day.

THERAPIST: Uh-huh. I hear sadness in your voice. It must have been very hard for you.

CLIENT: It was very hard. It still is. I think about her all the time. I keep thinking about her last minutes.

THERAPIST: I imagine it is difficult to be going through this.

Example 3

CLIENT: Well, just about 5 months ago, my best friend was killed in a car accident on her way to work. I basically figured out it was her by recognizing her car on the news because I was at home sick that day.

THERAPIST: Wow, it is awful to have a friend killed suddenly, but what an awful way to find out about it.

CLIENT: Yes, it was almost like I saw it. I called her cell phone right away, but a police officer answered and told me what had happened.

THERAPIST: How were you even able to process that information?

CLIENT: Well, I guess I fell apart. They asked me if I knew how to contact her family. I knew her mother's name and suspected it was in her cell phone.

THERAPIST: Were you alone during this time?

CLIENT: Yes, it was just me. I didn't think to call anyone. The police had been busy with the accident, I guess, and they hadn't had a chance to go through her cell phone. I couldn't even think about her mother's name, even though I knew it. Instead of me calling them, the police did.

THERAPIST: I can't imagine anyone would have been quick to think about those details under such shock.

CLIENT: I keep thinking about her last minutes, how scared she must have been.

THERAPIST: Of course, that seems like a pretty natural reaction to me.

While these examples are only illustrative, we have observed similar examples of therapist behavior. The last example intentionally shows the client giving more detail. When therapists are genuinely warm, clients are more likely to open up. It is easier to trust someone who comes across as legitimately caring than someone who is cold and aloof, or sounds like they are putting on an act. Feelings of warmth toward one's clients can be a challenge at times for even the most skillful therapists. At such times, we often suggest that clinicians go back to the basic treatment model and case conceptualization and ask themselves if there are important parts of the client's life context or history that they are missing. It also can be helpful to remember to practice being nonjudgmental and maintaining a problem-solving approach. When one finds a particular client to be disagreeable, hostile, or otherwise challenging, a therapist might recall the life course that conditioned the client to act in such a fashion. Subsequently remembering that many challenging clients are themselves finding life to be difficult can increase therapist empathy. When clients repeatedly challenge a therapist by not completing assignments or not fully engaging in therapy, the therapist can engage in problem solving with an attitude of curiosity about the contingencies influencing the client's behavior. Finally, having the ongoing support of a consultation team can be invaluable in maintaining warmth and genuine regard for one's clients, even when progress is slow.

Working to Reinforce Reports or Examples of Adaptive Behavior in Session

Clients may evidence adaptive behavior in sessions in a wide variety of ways. Some clients come to sessions well prepared to report verbally on active steps they took since the preceding session. They may report on a homework log or in conversation about social engagement, exercise, or work or home tasks. Other clients may show improved adaptive behavior during the actual session itself, such as by accomplishing things in session that demonstrate an increase in activation and engagement in the moment. For example, a client who typically stares at his shoes during the session may sit up and make eye contact more readily.

There is no prescription for how to reinforce reports or expressions of successful adaptive behaviors. Reinforcement is a tricky thing. We only know that a consequence or reward has been truly reinforcing when we see the sought behavior increase. Thus, therapists will need to make hunches based on their clinical expertise and knowledge of a particular client and what seems likely to reinforce positive change. For most clients, praise, genuine enthusiasm, and/or focused attention from the therapist are meaningful reinforcers. Attending to a client's activity chart, expressing "Wow, that is terrific!," or sitting up and warmly responding to the client are all examples of ways to reinforce a client. For example, a client who has been very inactive reported that he went to the market to buy fresh produce, and the therapist responded with genuine interest and curiosity, saying, "That is a change for you to go out to the store. Was it difficult? How did you get yourself to do it?" With such a response the therapist indicates that he or she sees the change, recognizes that this took effort on the client's part, and communicates the importance of this step through open-ended questions.

The key point is that the therapist must continually remain alert to reports or expressions of adaptive behavior and then consistently respond to them in some way that increases the likelihood that the client will continue such positive change. The skillful therapist does not let anything go by unnoticed. Any reports or expressions of adaptive behavior are opportunities for the therapist to selectively reinforce such behavior.

Summary

BA is a structured action-oriented therapy. Although the course of treatment is customized for each client, the structure of the treatment and the general approach of the therapist are consistent features. Table 3.2 provides a brief synopsis of the typical BA therapist's "style." Therapists structure treatment by collaboratively setting an agenda in each session, keeping in mind that activation is the key goal sought in therapy. Naturally the therapist begins by gathering a general understanding of the client's depression and the context in which it has arisen. Such an understanding sets the stage for developing treatment targets of behaviors to increase or decrease. The therapist accomplishes his or her work with the client while being validating and nonjudgmental and by making sure that the client understands treatment rationales and expectations. The therapist also works to reinforce the client's reports of or actual examples of adaptive behaviors during the therapy session. These elements of the treatment are considered necessary to effectively utilize the core assessment and activation strategies of BA that we discuss in the chapters that follow.

4

Identifying the Ingredients of the Behavioral Antidepressant

> Life consists of penetrating the unknown, and fashioning our
> actions in accord with the new knowledge thus acquired.
> —LEO TOLSTOY (1828–1910)

Alicia felt depressed daily and had a difficult time remembering whether there was a time when she had not felt so down every day. She always thought of herself as anxious, and her anxiety was troublesome but did not concern her as much as the deep depression in which she found herself. Her therapist, Beth, told her that they would work together to better understand the behaviors and situations that were associated with her depression as well as her anxiety and the difficulties in her relationships with other people. This sounded odd to her. She thought: "I feel terrible all the time—so, what's the point of identifying behaviors and situations? There is no time when I'm not depressed or worried." Beth suggested that there might be fluctuations in her mood that they could identify if they paid particular attention to her experiences each day. They began to talk in detail about earlier the same morning, before Alicia came to therapy. Beth asked about both Alicia's depressed mood and other emotions associated with various behaviors.

Alicia reported that she had walked to the grocery store, and, as she thought about it, she thought that perhaps her mood had improved ever so slightly. It was so brief, though, and she thought, "Does that really matter?" On the way home from the store, just a few minutes

60

later, she started feeling blue again, and once in her apartment it was like all of her energy had been drained out of her.

When Beth heard this, she asked Alicia whether she often felt worse when she was in her apartment. She wondered whether her apartment might be associated with all the painful things that had happened recently. As they talked more, Beth highlighted the types of activities in which Alicia engaged while in her apartment. They talked about how common it was for Alicia to lie on the bed drifting in and out of sleep or reading magazines that she described as "a stupid waste of time." Alicia acknowledged that she felt lonely and couldn't think of anything to do in her apartment.

She related a common occurrence that was particularly painful since she believed it had contributed to her friends' distancing themselves from her. Alicia had begun to dread the telephone ringing. Her phone had a caller identification computerized voice that reported the number or name of the caller. She had become so isolated that whenever the telephone rang Alicia would immediately become tense, dreading that one of her friends might call to check in or ask if she wanted to get together for a social event. If the caller ID was for a solicitor, she felt mildly annoyed but also relieved. If a friend called, she would listen for a moment to the computerized pronunciation of the name and then turn down the volume of the phone. When she couldn't hear the name, she felt slightly relieved, although she would not feel completely relieved until she had deleted any messages left, barely paying attention to what was said. Thinking to herself, "I'll call him or her back when I feel better," she'd settle into a nap and eventually wake up feeling even more empty and alone.

Introduction

BA is a highly idiographic approach to treatment. The treatment interventions are custom-tailored to each individual. The course of therapy for Alicia may look quite different from that of another client seeking treatment for depression. When providing such a flexible treatment, how is a therapist to determine what to do? How does Alicia's therapist begin to think about where to focus interventions and how to proceed with the process of change in order to help Alicia begin to lift her depression and stay well over time?

The bedrock of BA is the process of assessment. Through the

process of assessment, the BA therapist identifies how to individualize treatment. He or she figures out what is maintaining the problems that the client is experiencing and what will likely lead to improvement. The BA therapist identifies what treatment targets are likely to help alleviate a client's depression and help him or her move in the direction of important life goals. This chapter explains how to do just this. First, we describe what guides our assessment process, namely, an understanding of an individual client's goals. Second, we describe the "how-to" of doing assessment in BA. As in many behavioral therapies, assessment is ongoing and guides the therapist throughout the course of treatment.

Assessing Goals

The assessment process begins with exploring client goals. This is particularly important because BA is a short-term, action-oriented therapy, requiring that treatment goals be identified early in therapy. Overall, the goal of BA is to help clients experience greater contact with sources of reward in their lives and solve life problems. The specific goals, however, are highly individualized.

Assessing client goals requires collaboration between the client and therapist. Although the emphasis on activation is the hallmark of BA, therapists cannot just tell clients to get busy. In fact, most depressed individuals have already heard this advice or have told themselves to "Just do it!" thousands of times. We assume, however, that if they could simply get off the couch and get moving, they would have done so without the trouble and expense of seeking professional help. Thus, it's important to start treatment by asking "What does the client *want*?"

Many clients initially want to feel better. This is a reasonable desire for someone who is depressed, but it is difficult to achieve. In the behavioral model, it is activation and engagement in activities that are ultimately expected to have a positive impact on mood. Therefore, it is important to move rapidly from desired feelings to desired behaviors and personal goals. People can take many short-term steps to action in pursuit of a long-term goal. Engaging in the short-term goals may very well result in a feeling of accomplishment or enjoyment for the client. Regardless of how he or she feels, however, making steps toward a desired goal keeps the client moving forward and also improves the client's life situation.

Knowing what a client values may also help in identifying appropriate goals. Focusing on values can also be very helpful during stuck points, when clients face conflicting and competing goals. Hayes et al. (1999) differentiate values from goals, defining values as desired life consequences that provide one a sense of direction but that (unlike goals) cannot be intentionally attained or obtained. People can continually act according to their values, and they can pursue goals that are attainable along the way. The value held can move one's actions toward one goal or another. A focus on values is a primary undercurrent of behavioral treatments, such as acceptance and commitment therapy (ACT; Hayes et al., 1999). We recommend that therapists learn about the values work that is typically a part of ACT, as it can be easily integrated into BA. Dahl, Plumb, Stewart, and Lundgren (2009) highlight the importance of values work in therapy and provide strategies for doing so based on ACT. Through exploring goals and values, the therapist can develop an understanding of the kind of life a client would like to have, which in turn helps to shape how to individualize BA goals for a given client.

Take, for instance, the person who values being a good friend. He has been asked by his best friend to help move a heavy piece of furniture over the weekend to make room for visiting guests, and he is the only friend available to help. On Saturday, however, he wakes up feeling very depressed and lethargic and wants to stay at home and keep the shades drawn. He now has two competing and conflicting goals, the goal to help his friend in need and a competing goal of getting relief from the mood-dependent pressure to withdraw from the world for the day. If he acts according to what he values, he is more likely to choose to help his friend. It is then more likely that he will feel a little better at the end of the day and be less likely to withdraw further and become more depressed. In BA, it can be helpful to assess basic values and goals related to the domains of family, interpersonal relationships, work, and leisure. Derek Hopko, Carl Lejuez, and their colleagues also have developed a number of creative methods for assessing client goals and values. In their book on BA treatment for depression for cancer patients, Hopko and Lejuez (2007) provide a guide for clients to evaluate their goals and values in several domains.

The Basics of Behavioral Assessment

The third principle of BA guides the "how-to" of assessment in BA. This principle involves investigating clues and figuring out what is going to be antidepressant by noticing what precedes and what follows important behavior. People generally are unaware of the connections interlocking various situations, activities, and feelings. In the midst of depression, it can be even harder to recognize such relationships. The process of assessment in BA helps to provide data to both the clinician and the client regarding these important relationships. Detecting such relationships helps guide the identification of the behavioral targets of treatment that will lead to meeting treatment goals.

How does the therapist go about doing this? First, the therapist asks questions to *define and describe the key problems* that clients experience. Second, the therapist *assesses the cues and consequences* of client behaviors. Third, once the therapist has developed an understanding of the cues and consequences of specific instances of client behavior, the therapist begins to *assess patterns of behavior* that occur across time and settings. Often, understanding these patterns enables the therapist to know what to change to help alleviate the depression.

To conduct behavioral assessments productively, it is useful for BA therapists to understand the basic "ABCs" of behavior. To understand the *A,* it's important to appreciate that all behavior is contextual; that is, behavior happens in *particular* situations. We call these situations the "antecedents"—the *A.* The *B* refers to the "behavior" that we are seeking to understand. Often the *B*s are what bring people to therapy, such as fighting with partners, missing days at work, not being successful in finding a job, and so forth. We discuss in more detail shortly about how to define and describe the *B.* And, finally, all behaviors have some effects—these are the "consequences," the *C* (see Figure 4.1).

Defining and Describing Behavior

Let's start by talking about the *B*s. It is important to define and describe the primary problem behaviors clearly. When conducting behavioral assessments, therapists often need to ask a lot of questions about the behaviors of their clients in order to understand the behav-

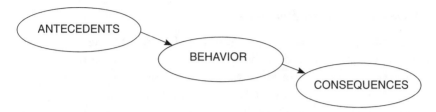

FIGURE 4.1. Functional analysis. Given certain antecedents (*A*), a behavior occurs (*B*), and the consequences (*C*) determine whether the behavior increases (i.e., is reinforced) or decreases (i.e., is punished).

iors in concrete terms. Often it is helpful to think about problems as behaviors that need to be either increased or decreased.

Behaviors to increase include those that are likely to bring a client into contact with positive reinforcement in the environment and to solve problems or improve the overall quality of life. These activities need to be increased because they bring reward into one's life, either through a sense of competence or pleasure, or solve problems. These behaviors can be increased via activity scheduling. We discuss this topic in more detail in Chapter 5. Another common behavior that needs to be increased is actively approaching problems and using problem solving. Often depressed clients come in with a host of problems that render them overwhelmed and stuck. As a coach, the therapist helps the client break tasks into smaller steps, prioritize, learn necessary skills, and make a commitment to tackle the problem.

Behaviors to decrease are those that make the client's life more difficult or interfere with managing one's needs; typically these are avoidance patterns. Such behaviors may include ruminating, engaging in behavior that is congruent with mood but counter to one's goal, or other escape or avoidance behavior, such as drinking. These behaviors often are maintained via negative reinforcement in that they tend to provide relief from an aversive circumstance or context in the short run but are often maladaptive in the long run.

Once the therapist has defined and described the problems, it is important to incorporate the third principle of identifying the antecedents and consequences of client behavior—the *A*'s and the *C*'s. As the therapist builds an understanding of specific instances of client behavior, he or she can also start to weave an understanding of important patterns of behavior that persist across settings and time.

Antecedents and Behaviors

The relationships between the A's and the B's are often very important in BA. Certain antecedents will increase the likelihood that certain behaviors will occur. In fact, we have often been conditioned to feel and think in certain ways under specific circumstances through the process of classical or respondent conditioning (Pavlov, 1927; Watson & Raynor, 1920; Wolpe, 1958). Respondent conditioning refers to the ways in which the normal pairing of events affects human behavior. Some events in our environment elicit responses without requiring special conditioning or training. For example, we have a startle reflex when we hear a loud noise. Other situations are relatively neutral but can become paired with intense feeling. For example, walking through a field is, for most people, a neutral event; if, however, an individual takes a long walk through a field that happens to be next to a military training area in which explosives are being set off, the individual may begin to feel mild dread when approaching an open field. This sense of dread would reflect the pairing of the unconditioned stimulus (loud noise) that elicits a startle response with the neutral stimulus of the field and can result in the field's taking on some of the anxiety-eliciting properties that loud noises bring about.

These types of relationships between A's and B's are often important in understanding our clients' experiences of depression. Jack provides a good example of this phenomenon. He grew up in a working-class family and was sent to an elite high school on a scholarship. During school, he observed that his well-dressed classmates seemed to have an easier time managing classes and social relationships. They also teased him occasionally for not being conversant with certain cultural references (such as the names of famous tennis players, who for Jack, a working-class kid, were less familiar). Jack's family had never traveled; so, he felt ashamed and conspicuous in classes when his peers would chat about having spent summers abroad. For him, the sight of well-dressed peers became a stimulus for negative thoughts about his failures and shortcomings. This conditioned response persisted into adulthood and became evident as he moved into a management-level position in his company. As he began to attend meetings with senior management, the mere presence of accomplished colleagues elicited anxiety and negative thoughts. He had difficulty speaking up in meetings even though he had significant contributions to make; on more than one occasion, as he sat quietly pondering solutions to problems to himself, one of his colleagues would express precisely the same idea that he had. His discomfort around "upper-class people" was classically conditioned early in his school years and continued to exert influence over his behavior. Over time, Jack began to avoid these meetings, and his work performance suffered, initiating a cycle of withdrawal and depression.

In such ways, our feelings, thoughts, and actions occur under certain conditions in certain environments. Often the feelings we experience have been conditioned through the process of experiencing distress or pleasure under similar conditions (respondent conditioning), and then our behaviors under those conditions are maintained through the consequences. Melanie, whose 3-month-old infant died suddenly 2 years ago, experienced crippling grief when asked to hold the newborn baby of a friend. For Melanie, the antecedent of being close to an infant increased the likelihood of feeling pain. Like Jack and Melanie, many of our clients have had various conditions paired with painful feelings earlier in their life experiences. Often our clients have lost sight of these contextual factors and their profound effect on their feelings. One of the jobs of the BA therapist is to begin to disentangle the relationships between antecedents and important behaviors.

Behaviors and Consequences

The relationships between the B's and the C's are heavily emphasized in BA. When a behavior is followed by a consequence that increases it, we say the behavior has been reinforced. When an action results in the attainment of something desired, that action has been positively reinforced. When someone introduces herself to a new neighbor and the neighbor responds by saying how delighted she is to meet her, and they have subsequent conversations from time to time, we know that greeting the neighbor has been positively reinforced.

We also learn by avoiding what we don't want. When a behavior results in the removal of something noxious to the organism, that behavior is likely to occur again under similar conditions. We say that the behavior has been negatively reinforced. For instance, Jack responded to his distress at management meetings by staying in bed late and avoiding such meetings as much as possible. When he did so, his feelings of discomfort were reduced; thus, staying in bed and going late to meetings were negatively reinforced. Unfortunately, over time, Jack's behavior also maintained the conditioned response of discomfort with his coworkers rather than being replaced by behavior that countered such a response by having Jack state his ideas and provide him an opportunity to experience a sense of accomplishment and mastery.

Behavior can also be punished. Whenever the consequence of a behavior decreases the likelihood of its happening again under similar circumstances, whether the consequence is something bad happening or something good being taken away, we say the behavior has been punished. Thus, if Jack were to begin speaking up at meetings and a senior colleague responded with a mocking tone, it is likely that Jack's assertiveness would be punished and therefore less likely to occur again in the future. Similarly, if Jack spoke up and the result was that his choice office location was assigned to someone else shortly thereafter, it is likely that his speaking up would be similarly decreased.

The function of a behavior refers to the particular consequences, such as reinforcement or punishment that follows a behavior. In BA, we are very interested in the function of a behavior. In fact, we are more interested in a behavior's function than its form, or the way it appears to us. For example, in her engaging popular book on behaviorism and positive training techniques, Amy Sutherland (2008) points out that, although humans want to express affection by giving a hug, to many animals being held tightly means it is about to be eaten. Thus, the function of a hug for an animal is to create terror—even though, to humans, the form or the way the behavior "looks" suggests building a bond of affection.

Darren provides a good example of the importance of the function over the form of a behavior. He had been depressed for 2 years prior to coming to therapy. His family history included the death of his younger sister when he was 15. When Darren was riding bikes with his sister, who was 11 years old, he crossed an intersection with her following, and just as she was in the middle of the street a car made a hasty turn, hitting her, and she died 5 days later in the hospital. Following this death, Darren's mother suffered from depression during much of his remaining high school years. There were no other children in the family, and Darren's father was a busy contractor who stayed late nights at work after Amy's death and rarely spent time with Darren. The family had a good deal of money and sent Darren to a prestigious college, from which he graduated with honors. He then began a successful career in upper management. At the age of 38 he was successful, had a happy marriage, and had one child, a daughter.

Darren's depression began when his daughter was 8 years old, and followed the death of his uncle from a heart attack. Darren had been close to his uncle, having spent summers on his uncle's farm from the age of 16 until he went away to college. Darren's daughter was 10 at the time he entered therapy. Despite his depression, he spent a great deal of time playing with his daughter. They particularly enjoyed outdoor activities like hiking, softball, and swimming. Darren and his wife took their daughter bike riding on local trails. They always went riding as a family and made it a point to ride on the trails every weekend when the sun was out. To any observer this looked like productive family-oriented behavior that would be helpful for improving his mood and well-being, and good for his daughter and family life as well. However, Darren did not let his daughter ride her bike at any other time. He and his wife argued a great deal about how much independence they would allow their daughter to have. She was forbidden from riding on public streets or even from riding with the families of some of her friends. The weekend riding came to be a slavish routine that allowed Darren to avoid the anxious feelings about his daughter's independence and also to avoid the grief he reexperienced about his sister whenever he worried about his daughter's being on city streets with her bike. While the form of Darren's actions looked like he was doing "active good dad" behavior, the bike riding actually functioned to allay his fears about his daughter's having an accident and served to diminish his feelings of guilt over his sister's death and his mother's subsequent depression. Thus, the behavior functioned as subtle avoidance of negative affect triggered by the similarity of this situation to his sister's accident many years before.

In BA, we look for the ways that behavior makes sense in the given context. We look for the situations that elicit behavior and the ways in which behavior is reinforced. In other words, the most important aspects of any behavior to understand are the situations in which it occurs and the functions that it serves. With these basics under your belt, let's turn to how a therapist actually goes about doing assessment in BA.

Assessment How-To: The Activity Chart

The activity chart is the primary tool used to conduct assessments in BA. We begin activity monitoring by familiarizing clients with the purposes of doing this. We normally tell them that the chart, or log, provides the best means for us to get a sense of what their lives really look like outside of the therapy hour. We encourage clients, rather than trusting to their memory, to record daily activities as close to the time that they occurred as possible. We urge them to act like scientists, examining their lives in detail, and to closely examine and record even the small things that they might otherwise think are unimportant.

There are standard activity charts that are typically used in CBT, and we use these frequently. At the same time, however, we allow considerable flexibility in how clients monitor themselves. Essentially, clients can use whatever form is useful to them. Some clients record activities in electronic data devices, others write lists on Post-it notes or on calendars. The exact form is less important than the data gathered. As our friend and colleague Steve Hollon noted, "We would even accept information recorded on a napkin" if it helped the client keep track of an activity and mood. The standard charts typically have very little room for writing (see Appendices 1b–1f). The client only needs to jot down a few words as a reminder about the activity rather than write extensive notes about individual activities.

Activity monitoring basically involves having the client write down activities in which he or she has engaged during the day for each day of the week prior to the next session. Clients can record their behaviors in a number of ways.

1. *Hour-by-hour monitoring.* This method will provide the most information and is more likely to be accurate since the client records his or her activity and associated mood each hour as the activities occur. The client completes a monitoring chart hourly and keeps track of all waking hours during the day, every day. This level of detail can be difficult for some clients. Although it provides the therapist with the most information, it is often impractical and in our experience is very rarely used successfully by all but the most detail-oriented clients. We encourage clients to record the activities as

closely to their actual occurrence as possible, and at the same time we understand that few clients will carry their chart with them and write down their activity each and every hour throughout the day. Clients also may elect to record at this level of detail only for selected days prior to the next session.

2. *Monitoring blocks of time during the day.* This easier method involves monitoring in blocks of time. Although the client is still asked to record activities for each hour of the day, the recording takes place periodically during the day, and the client is asked to recall the preceding 3–4 hours and record what he or she was doing and feeling during that time period. For example, a client might record his morning activities during the lunch hour, afternoon activities at dinnertime, and evening activities just prior to retiring for bed. Although this method is easier to use and is probably how most clients actually complete the monitoring, it may be less reliable since it involves more recall. Seriously depressed clients may have difficulty recalling subtle mood shifts that occurred during earlier hours and thus may not keep a detailed account of mood. Nevertheless, this method can still provide the therapist and the client with important information that helps to guide the work of BA.

3. *Time-sampling procedures.* Another way to gather information from clients is to ask them to do time-sampling procedures, which is a way to do spot checks on their behavior. When setting the self-monitoring assignment, set specific hours during which the client will monitor his or her activity ahead of time. For example, a client may be asked to record activities and mood between 1 P.M. and 3 P.M. on Monday, between 8 A.M. and 10 A.M. on Wednesday, between 6 P.M. and 8 P.M. on Friday, and between noon and 2 P.M. on Sunday. It is very important that there be a variety in the times set aside for monitoring and equally important that the client include daytime and evening periods and also include a weekend day or evening. This approach provides a better sample of the variety of activities and moods and gives the clinician and client a better picture of various contexts that may influence the client's mood. The times during which the client will self-monitor and record should be written down either directly on the activity chart—perhaps marked for emphasis with a colored highlight—or in an electronic scheduler if available.

What to Monitor

There are several elements to record in an Activity Chart: the activity, one's mood or feelings at the time of the activity, and the intensity of mood. Clients can also record whether or not they felt pleasure or a sense of accomplishment when engaging in an activity. Each of these components is discussed in detail below.

Monitoring Activities

When instructing clients about recording activity, it is often helpful to guide them in finding a balance between recording too little and too much. The client does not need to record so much in each hour that the information is unwieldy but needs to record enough so that the therapist and client both know what is happening. Often, as clients begin monitoring, they will record global entries that include large blocks of time. For instance, they may write "at work" for 8 hours, with their mood described as "bored" and rated as an "8" for the entire time. The problem with such entries is that they miss valuable information that comes from noticing variability. When one has had a "bad day" at work, it is not usually the case that every minute of every hour was bad. The activity of being "at work" is actually a combination of many more specific activities, and often these are important to record. Perhaps a chat with a colleague in the coffee room was enjoyable; and while reading endless e-mail may, in fact, have been boring, an e-mail about an upcoming project may have been less boring than an e-mail about a new requirement for clocking hours. While it is unrealistic to expect that a client will record a shift in mood for each e-mail read, it is reasonable to expect that recording feeling "engaged" during the hour in which the coffee room conversation occurred and "bored" during the hour when one was reading e-mail will provide more meaningful information than simply writing "bored" for the entire workday.

We urge clients to monitor themselves at this level of specificity because mood changes reflected on the chart help to identify the activities that are associated with depressed moods and improved moods. Quantifying this variability helps us to figure out what activities to increase or decrease. In this way, monitoring helps identify specific targets for treatment. For example, it is valuable to know that

Alicia's mood is more positive when she reads a book on gardening on a Saturday morning than when she reads a magazine on Monday evening. Such change signals that something is going on there. Often people experience momentary shifts in mood in one direction or the other that can help to guide future activation plans. It can require coaching and practice to begin to notice such subtle changes in mood with different activities.

For some clients, it is also important to record internal activities, such as ruminating. For instance, a client may record "talking to a neighbor" and also record a mood of "despair." With that amount of information the therapist may wonder if there is something stressful about the neighbor. Upon further inquiry, however, the therapist may learn that the client was talking with the neighbor about their respective lawns and during this conversation was ruminating about how he used to enjoy his lawn but no longer cares now that he's depressed. In this case, it would have been important to record "ruminating" as a behavior on the activity chart that would more accurately portray the pattern of behavior (in this case, rumination) that is connected with despair. Talking to the neighbor is certainly an important part of the client's experience, but the heart of the matter in this example is what is occurring privately for the client.

Monitoring Mood or Emotion

When orienting clients to recording their moods and emotions and the intensity of them, it is helpful to begin with a single dimensional scale of mood, such as depressed mood ranging from a "1" for "not at all intense" to a "10" for "very intense." As clients develop greater familiarity with the Activity Chart and with attention to their emotional experience, they can be encouraged to record a range of specific emotions (e.g., sad, angry, happy, ashamed, disgusted, afraid, and so forth) and the intensity of each emotion. Some clients experience difficulty in identifying specific emotions, which presents an opportunity for BA therapists to provide education and skills training practice. For more extensive information on the identification of specific emotions, therapists are encouraged to consult the emotion regulation skills training module of the skills training manual for dialectical behavior therapy (Linehan, 1993), which defines sadness, happiness, fear, anger, shame, disgust, and surprise.

Monitoring Mastery and Pleasure

As an alternative to monitoring mood, clients can also record the experience of mastery or pleasure associated with activities (Beck et al., 1979). Mastery is the sense of accomplishment experienced, and pleasure is the feeling of enjoyment that accompanies an activity. Rating these dimensions provides a way to track activities that are more or less functional—namely, those that result in a sense of mastery and/or pleasure. Intensity of mastery and pleasure is also recorded on a 10-point scale, with "1" indicating "low" mastery or pleasure and "10" indicating "high" mastery or pleasure (see Appendix 1d).

Monitoring Intensity

It is important to record intensity so that subtle changes on the activity chart can be captured. Consider a client who only reports "sad" as a feeling on his activity chart. His therapist will want the client to indicate times when he was more or less sad so that she can help him to begin examining activities associated with shifts in mood. It is often valuable to help clients anchor the endpoints of the intensity scales with real activities in their lives. For example, when Alicia's therapist first introduced mood monitoring, she worked with Alicia to identify activities that were associated with the high and low ends of the intensity scale. In recording mood, reading a popular entertainment magazine was associated with feeling down at a low level of "3," on a scale of 0–10, whereas listening to her answering machine messages received a rating of "10." Similarly, on a mastery scale, reading the magazine provided a minimal sense of mastery and was rated a "1," whereas reading a chapter in a book about gardening received a mastery rating of "10." When rating intensity, therapists may find that some clients don't like to use numerical ratings. It is sensible in such cases to use ratings on dimensions indicated by words, for example, "a little" to "a great deal." In other cases, clients may even use some other symbol to indicate his or her rating.

Ultimately, the particular monitoring system is not as important as ensuring that a clear method has been devised that will provide data about the effects of specific activities. The connection between specific activities and how the client is feeling and functioning is the ultimate target for all types of monitoring. As long as the monitoring is always focused on activity and the context of the activity, the monitoring will be useful. Prior to sending the client home with an activity monitoring chart, the therapist can ask the client to record some information on the chart for the few hours immediately preceding therapy and the therapy session itself and note what actions took place and what feelings were present.

Reviewing Activity Monitoring

Once the client has completed the monitoring assignment between therapy sessions, the therapist will spend a good portion of the following session reviewing the chart. When reviewing the activity chart, the therapist can either read it aloud or ask the client to do so. Initially it is good to begin the discussion by asking the client what he or she generally learned from the monitoring. The client may have noticed behavior patterns or clues to the links between activity and mood. The therapist will then review the chart along with the client to consider other patterns that can be discussed with the client and can then be used to generate treatment targets.

Useful Questions to Facilitate the Review

There are five questions that can guide therapists during the review, which often help to identify the specific activities or behaviors that are serving to maintain depression. Although it is not necessary to ask all of the questions, keeping them in mind can help to better understand the client's behavior patterns.

1. What are the connections between the client's activities and moods? These types of questions are used to generate hypotheses about the contingencies at work in maintaining the client's depression. It is important to notice, first of all, where the shifts in mood occur. Clients and therapists may start this discussion by looking for patterns of behavior associated with particular moods. A question like "Can you tell me what you noticed from recording this week?" can be helpful in getting started. Understanding the behaviors that make the client more or less depressed as well as the contexts in which moods change is essential. Beth, the therapist working with Alicia, made note of contextual factors like the fact that Alicia felt blue when she was working in the community pea patch garden one day and happy on another. What qualities of the two activities are related to

the differences in mood? Taking particular notice of activities that are associated with more positive mood will yield valuable data that will suggest behaviors to increase.

BETH: I notice on Monday that you have written "working in garden" and you have written that your mood was "blue," whereas on Tuesday you have "working in garden" and you've recorded your mood as "happy." What was different about those two days?

ALICIA: Well, it's not really "my" garden. I participate in a "pea patch" that I share with other people. I guess I was more down on Monday.

BETH: Did that start before you began to work in the pea patch?

ALICIA: I don't really think so. What did I write earlier?

BETH: Oh, yes, I see here that just about an hour before you wrote that you made a cup of tea after work and you were feeling "contented." What do you think happened that made that shift when you were working in the garden?

ALICIA: I think it was just the time of day. It was starting to get a little dark out, and I think the gloom and, if I remember correctly, the drizzle made me just feel kind of sad. I wanted to enjoy the garden, but I couldn't shake the gloominess, and feeling like I had to hurry before the sun went down completely. I think the feeling that it was especially dark inside when I went back to the apartment also influenced how I rated the mood.

BETH: So, it was really important that the weather affected your mood, and especially the gloom.

ALICIA: Yes, but also that I really dread going back into the apartment if I've not enjoyed a little bit of sunshine. Tuesday was better. I think I went out a little earlier, and the weather was better. I think I even stayed out longer.

BETH: Yes, you've actually got "working in the garden" recorded over a couple of hours on Tuesday. So, were you were saddened on Monday by the gloom?

ALICIA: No, by how much I hate my apartment. I usually feel really good when I'm in the garden. I'm usually there by myself, for the most part. On Monday there were a few other people there, and they were kind of loud. I got really quiet. Sometimes I sing to myself when I am in the garden, and that feels good. I also tend to take a look around at what is growing, but these other people made me feel a little annoyed and I just stayed in one little spot.

BETH: Was this different than on Tuesday?

ALICIA: Oh, yes. On Tuesday I was the only person there for the first 20 minutes. Then another woman came along, but she was friendly and quiet. She said "Hi" and primarily worked in a different part of the garden. She did come by and commented on how nicely a few plants were doing, and we chatted a bit about how lovely the garden was.

BETH: So, although you were working in the garden on both days, when you were just stuck in the gloom, silent, avoiding the loud people on Monday, you felt blue. But when the weather was a little better, it was earlier, and you engaged in conversation with the woman about the garden, you felt happy. The situations were slightly different, and in each situation something different was required of you, right? On Monday you needed to finish quickly because it was getting dark, and also you were a bit hampered by the noisy people. On Tuesday you could take more time, and having someone pleasant around required you to actually engage a little.

ALICIA: Yes.

BETH: This is really good to see how these different situations, and the different actions associated with them, affect your mood.

Likewise, asking what activities are associated with more negative mood allows the therapist to discuss the problems with these activities with the client. They won't necessarily become behaviors to decrease, since the therapist will first need to understand what it is about the activities that are associated with worsened mood. In the example of Alicia in the pea patch, one would not want to suggest she stop going on Mondays and only go to the pea patch on Tuesdays. Beth might suggest, however, behaviors in the garden for Alicia to increase, such as looking at plants, singing to herself, and having brief conversations with others. Behaviors to decrease might be ruminating about her apartment, avoiding people, and staying in one spot rather than looking around the whole garden. Clearly, however, there is a lot more for Alicia and Beth to learn together. Beth may want to ask a number of follow-up questions, such as: What does Alicia talk about with others in the garden? What are typical responses of others who share the pea patch? Beth might ask similar questions of Alicia's interactions with a variety of people. Are there ways that she inadvertently punishes people's conversational behavior? Does she avoid having lengthy conversations with people and thus give the impression that she is not very approachable?

Looking at the behaviors associated with shifts in mood can also yield other important information about clients, like whether there are interruptions in normal routines, such as sleeping, eating, and working. It may be an effective initial treatment strategy to target routine regulation. Parents and BA therapists know that it is difficult to tackle life's problems without adequate sleep or nutrition. Avoiding work can lead to multiple problems that can worsen the client's depression. Avoidance in general is a primary pattern that is assessed and treated in BA. Thus, we use activity monitoring to assess the second type of question.

2. What is the client's overall mood, and what are the specific emotions experienced throughout the week? Often clients are engaged in a variety of activities but experience a narrow range of emotions. Using an activity and emotion chart, on which clients are asked to record various moods, the therapist can observe the range of emotions reported. When clients have reported different emotions throughout the week, the therapist has an opportunity to review the connections between particular activities and emotions in order to develop initial hypotheses about possible activities to increase or decrease. When clients have reported only one or two emotions, it can be helpful for the therapist to do additional assessment. A few possible reasons may be that the client lacks skill in identifying and articulating how he or she feels at any given moment. These and many other possibilities can be explored.

3. Has there been a disruption in the client's routine? Reviewing activity monitoring charts provides a glimpse of a client's daily or weekly routine. A therapist may be concerned when he or she sees radical changes in the times a client goes to bed in the evening or wakes up in the morning, or when the client records highly variable mealtimes from day to day. When clients are depressed, they may get out of their normal routines. Thus, another focus of BA is to help clients regulate their routines (Martell et al., 2001) to provide them with a sense of normalcy. The increased structure and predictability

also can be helpful in keeping clients organized and on task. When routines are severely disrupted, it can feel overwhelming at times—for example, when a job is lost and one's naturally structured day suddenly fills up with excessive free time. Consider the typical relief one feels to be home, back at the office, or sleeping in one's own bed following a busy business trip or even a vacation. Getting back to a normal routine can be comforting, and the disruption in routine when an individual is depressed may deprive him or her of that comfort. We do not suggest that depression results from the disruption of one's routine, but the possible benefits of helping depressed clients maintain a regular routine is partially supported by literature suggesting that dysregulation of social routines contributes to the onset of major depressive episodes or manic episodes in persons with bipolar spectrum disorders (Shen, Alloy, Abramson, & Sylvia, 2008).

4. What avoidance patterns are present? It is a good thing to know what the client is avoiding in his or her life. Sometimes avoidance is very clear-cut, as when a client is avoiding getting up in the morning. Other times it is more subtle, as when a client is avoiding situations that trigger feelings of shame (e.g., Jack skipping management meetings at work). It is important to know what is getting in the way of engaging in and enjoying life since avoidance leads to passivity, that is, problems go unsolved or continue to get larger. The activity chart can suggest the problems in the client's life that need to be solved. For example, when a client consistently records a negative mood whenever he or she engages in a task for work, it may be worth exploring whether the client's job is a poor fit for him or her. The relationships between avoidance patterns and moods can also be tricky because clients sometimes feel better when they are avoiding. In fact, for many people, this is what motivates more avoidance. Either they feel relief, or they actually feel good. Consider this example of Alicia, who felt relieved by avoiding a social event:

ALICIA: I don't know, I just didn't go to my friend's first book club meeting even though I'd planned to go.

BETH: Was this a last-minute decision not to go?

ALICIA: Yes, I was even thinking about getting dressed, even was trying to pick an outfit.

BETH: What happened then?

ALICIA: I started to feel really bad about how I never say the right things about the book in a book club. Others are so much smarter. I felt kind of stupid. All of my insecurities just came over me.

BETH: Has that happened before when you've attended a book club?

ALICIA: Sometimes, but people are usually nice, and I knew my friend had only invited nice people. I just couldn't get myself to go the other night. I felt ashamed of myself and guilty that I've seemed to squander my life and not spend the time reading and getting to know more about the world so that I could also be articulate. When I decided not to go, I was relieved, and I was happy to stay at home.

A further complicating factor about avoidance that therapists need to keep in mind is that clients who use mind-altering substances to avoid feeling down often are quite successful at making themselves feel rather good. Paying attention to the function of behavior, therapists need to know whether recreational use of substances is a social behavior with few adverse consequences or if it is a way of escaping negative feelings and at risk for exacerbation. With all of this contextual information, the therapist is ready to focus on the fifth type of question.

5. Where should one start making changes? Looking over a client's activity chart, even after just a week of monitoring, can suggest behaviors that are effective candidates for maximizing change. When we know what activities are associated with improvements in mood, we then need to know which activities will be easier to increase when the client is feeling unmotivated. Likewise, we want to know which of the activities that are associated with negative mood or avoidance the client can most easily begin to decrease. Once identified, decreases in avoidance behavior can be planned step by step, beginning with decreasing the amount, such as reducing drinking four glasses of wine a night to three, or decreasing the time spent in a mindless avoidance activity. Asking a client who spends nearly 5 hours each day playing computer games as a distraction and avoidance technique to replace this activity with more productive behavior and reduce computer game time to 30 minutes a day is likely to prove unsuccessful, at least initially. Instead, developing a plan collaboratively with the client to determine a reasonable reduction in computer game time—say, reducing it by 10 minutes daily for two nights, then another 10 minutes on the third and fourth days, and so on—may

be more likely to succeed. The same gradualist principle is true for behaviors associated with negative mood. Beth noticed that Alicia had reported feeling slightly better when she walked to the grocery store but that her mood soon worsened. However, this first step was considered a behavior to increase.

BETH: Alicia, do you think that it was the walk or the grocery store that made you feel slightly better?

ALICIA: Probably the walk. I usually just drive to the store. I don't particularly like shopping.

BETH: So you walked once, your mood improved, but then your mood worsened. What do you think might happen if you walked more times during the upcoming week?

ALICIA: I don't know. It is a little lonely to walk alone. I think that was why I felt badly.

BETH: Do you have a friend who might walk with you?

ALICIA: I could ask someone if they wanted to take a little walk around the neighborhood. My next-door neighbor has invited me several times to do that. She wants to get more exercise.

BETH: I think that is a great idea. It will be interesting to see if walking with someone makes you feel better. When might you do that?

ALICIA: I could ask her if she'd like to walk tomorrow. I can call her this afternoon.

BETH: What if she says she's unavailable? Would you give her a few times from which to choose?

ALICIA: I could do that, I guess. I also could walk once with her and once alone and just see how it feels.

BETH: Okay, let's decide some possible days for doing that. You can set your time to walk alone. The walk with the neighbor will depend on her schedule; so, let's consider several options.

Assessing Risk

Finally, when needed, the therapist will assess risk. Therapists working with depressed clients always need to consider the possibility of suicidal ideation and actions. If therapists routinely use a self-report depression inventory, the therapist should always note the client's response to suicide items. If the client reports suicidal ideation, a safety assessment must be conducted. In cases where the therapist is not using self-report measures, he or she should ask clients about suicidal thoughts or plans. A risk assessment should be routine during initial interviews with depressed clients. Such questions should be asked in a straightforward manner. A therapist might say something like: "It is not uncommon for people to want to escape their depression and to have thoughts of hurting themselves. Do you ever have thoughts about wanting to die or to hurt or kill yourself?" If the client states that suicidal thoughts are present, the therapist must assess whether the client actively thinks about the desire to be dead or, alternatively, merely considers suicide as a possible escape from his or her emotional distress, as the two possibilities present differently. When a client no longer wishes to be in the world and may be making plans to end his or her life, the therapist should be especially alert to the imminent danger of suicide. This is a far more dangerous scenario than when the client doesn't have an active desire to die but simply cannot think of any other solution to the problem of his or her depression, and passively thinking about death provides relief from stress. In either case, therapists must not be cavalier about the client's reports of suicidal ideation and should carefully assess whether or not the client is in immediate danger. Given that approximately 15% of severely depressed patients die by suicide, it is essential to assess the nature of the client's ideation, plans, intent, access to means, and potential deterrents. There are excellent texts on managing suicidal behavior by experts in this area that provide essential reading for all therapists working with depressed clients (e.g., Bongar, 2002; Jobes, 2006). Other risks that need to be assessed are the presence of weapons in the household, medications that may be used for self-harm, and other means for hurting oneself or others to which the client may have access.

Making an Effective Choice of Activities

As we've discussed, there are two general types of activities or behaviors that a BA therapist can target to alleviate depression. There are activities that improve the mood and life context, which are targets to increase. There are also activities that maintain a depressed mood or that make life worse and so should be decreased. Clients may express a preference for specific activities to increase or decrease. Given the variety of behaviors to target, it is best to work on behaviors that will have the quickest impact. When we discuss the BA model with clients, we often point out that the place to begin is by targeting the behaviors that temporarily ease distress—albeit not sufficiently to relieve them totally of depression—that is, the "secondary problems." We attempt to break the short-term cycle of depression-prone behaviors prior to helping clients to make longer-term changes that may be more time-consuming. For example, it is likely to have a greater impact on a client's mood to increase physical activity and social contacts prior to having the client engage in the longer-term goal of finding a better job.

Putting It All Together

Figure 4.2 is a sample of Alicia's activity monitoring chart. (Blank forms of activity charts can be found in Appendix 1.) Alicia recorded her entire day on Monday and portions of her day on Tuesday, Wednesday, Thursday, and Saturday. Look through the activity chart, and ask yourself the questions discussed in this chapter. Before reading on, take some time to review the activity chart and try to answer the following questions:

- What activity–mood relationships do you notice?
- What general emotions are reported in the chart?
- Where are there routine interruptions?
- What avoidance patterns may be interfering with her functioning?
- What behaviors may be targets to increase or decrease?

What to Notice in Alicia's Activity Chart

Let's take a look at Alicia's activity chart for some possible behavioral patterns and questions that a therapist might want to ask to understand these patterns in more detail. Alicia is spending many hours in bed and sleeping late most mornings. This seems like an important behavior that the therapist might want to spend some time seeking to define and describe in more detail. For instance, the therapist would want to ask her if this is consistent with the other days that were not

	Mon.	Tues.	Wed.	Thurs.	Fri.	Sat.	Sun.
7:00 A.M.	Asleep		Asleep	Asleep			
8:00 A.M.	In bed Sad - 10		Asleep	Asleep			
9:00 A.M.	In bed Sad - 10		In bed Dread - 8	Asleep			
10:00 A.M.	In bed Irritated - 10 Sad - 8	Work Miserable!!	In bed Dread - 8	Asleep			
11:00 A.M.	Driving to work Anxious - 4		Showering P = 1 M = 1	Asleep		Reading Gardening Content -6 M = 10	
12:00 P.M.	Updating website Bored - 6 Sad - 7 M - 0 P - 0		Driving to work Upset - 10			In yard, pulling weeds Content - 6 M - 10	
1:00 P.M.	Same						
2:00 P.M.	Same						
3:00 P.M.	Same						
4:00 P.M.	Driving home Relieved - 8						
5:00 P.M.	Eating salad Bored - 8 P - 1						
6:00 P.M.	Magazines Down 3 M - 1						
7:00 P.M.	Checking voice mail Down 10						
8:00 P.M.	TV Sad - 9 M - 0					Dinner with Ellen Relieved M = 9 P = 5	
9:00 P.M.	Same						
10:00 P.M.	Same						
11:00 P.M.	In bed						
12:00 A.M.	Asleep		Tossing and turning in bed				

FIGURE 4.2. Alicia's activity and emotion monitoring chart.

recorded. She also spends a great deal of time lying in bed in the late mornings when she is not sleeping, another pattern of behavior. Consider the following dialogue:

BETH: Alicia, can you tell me a little more about sleeping late in the mornings?

ALICIA: Well, I feel really tired and just stay asleep, or just stay in bed.

BETH: Is there a difference in how you feel when you sleep late and then awaken, like on Thursday, compared to when you are awake but staying in bed? You did the former on Thursday, but on Monday and Wednesday you were awake but didn't get out of bed.

ALICIA: I guess when I sleep late I feel tired when I finally get up, but after I have some coffee or a shower I typically feel a little better. When I stay in bed I just feel continually exhausted.

BETH: Does it matter when you get to bed at night?

ALICIA: Not really. I sometimes feel like I can sleep all of the time.

BETH: Does the quality of your sleep matter?

ALICIA: Yes, on those days when I sleep in late, it is often because I feel like I've tossed and turned most of the night. When I just stay in bed, it is usually that I just can't face the day.

Beth has begun to discover some important differences in the function of being in bed late. She also has discovered that Alicia has some occasional difficulties getting refreshing sleep. These differences between sleeping late because she has had a bad night and staying in bed because she is avoiding her day will lead to different activation strategies. These will be discussed in more detail in the next chapter.

What to Target after Reviewing the Activity Chart

A therapist may notice so many problems in Alicia's activities that it is difficult to know where to start. This is often how our clients feel as well. It is like being in a room with five doors to open: which door will lead to where we want to go most quickly? As we've noted previously, the key to understanding what is going to be antidepressant lies in observing what precedes and what follows a behavior. Consider some of the consequences of Alicia's behavior of staying in bed for long periods. All of these times are associated with painful feelings such as sadness and dread. The therapist may want to ask directly about these potential emotional consequences of staying in bed for hours.

When Beth inquired about her dread, Alicia said she dreaded going to work and the boredom of her job. Beth then asked about Tuesday, when Alicia simply wrote, "Work, Miserable!!" This is an example of a client writing too little on the activity chart, thus requiring the therapist to ask more specific questions to define the problem. Alicia said she felt like she had reached her limit and felt desperate all day to find a new job. When Beth asked if she had been looking for a new job, Alicia replied, "No, not for several months."

Beth hypothesized that a behavior to decrease would be lying in bed in the mornings. In order to do that, it would be important to increase some other activities that would replace lying in bed. Look at the activity chart for clues as to what these might be. Alicia felt content when she was reading or gardening. While it may be difficult for Alicia to jump out of bed and work in her garden or rush off to work, it might be reasonable for her to begin a morning routine of getting out of bed, fixing a cup of coffee, and reading a few pages of a good book.

Alicia felt relieved when she drove home from work on Monday. She had left work early that day, after having arrived around 11:30 A.M. This was an example of avoidance behavior. She continued to engage in avoidance by reading magazines and felt down—another behavior to decrease. It might be useful to design a plan for staying at work and engaging in a useful task rather than heading home to mindlessly rummage through magazines. Checking her voice mail also made her feel "down." It would be unwise to assume that this is a behavior to decrease, however. The reason Alicia felt down when she checked her voice mail was that the message was from a friend, Ellen, who, despite Alicia's absence, was still trying to maintain their friendship. Note that on Saturday Alicia actually had dinner with Ellen. She felt relieved and had a strong sense of mastery. Her relief was in the fact that she'd stopped avoiding at least one friend. Notice also that this occurred after she had done some reading and gardening, pulling some weeds in the yard. In fact, she had called Ellen from her cell phone and invited her to dinner right after she'd pulled her last weed. In BA we often tell clients that lethargy breeds lethargy and activity breeds activity. This appeared to be the case on Saturday with Alicia. Increasing contact with her friends may be a promising behavior to focus on that exemplifies the principle of aiming for behavior that is naturally reinforced. It also accords with such other BA principles as taking a problem-solving approach and initiating the change with small increases in approach behavior. Notice how the small changes Alicia made on Saturday resulted in a positive change in her mood. As her coach, Beth would now begin the process of helping her to plan activities that would more consistently result in either improved mood or bettering her life situation.

TABLE 4.1. Basics of Identifying Treatment Targets

- Define and describe the key problems the client experiences.
- Assess patterns of behavior.
- Use functional analysis—assessing the antecedent situations, behaviors, and consequences of behavior under typical conditions.
- Utilize the activity chart and other self-monitoring strategies.
- Monitor activities.
- Monitor mood and emotion.
- Monitor mastery and pleasure.
- Monitor intensity.
- Identify routine disruptions and avoidance patterns.
- Assess client risk.
- Collaboratively choose activities that are likely to break the depressive cycle.
- Identify initial steps for making changes.

From *Behavioral Activation for Depression: A Clinician's Guide* by Christopher R. Martell, Sona Dimidjian, and Ruth Herman-Dunn. Copyright 2010 by The Guilford Press. Permission to photocopy this table is granted to purchasers of this book for personal use only (see copyright page for details). Purchasers may download a larger version of this table from the book's page on The Guilford Press website.

Summary

As a BA therapist, you must always keep your eye on the prize of activation—always alert to what is going to make it more or less likely

5

Activity Scheduling
and Structuring

Have a bias toward action—let's see something happen now.
You can break that big plan into small steps and take the first
step right away.
—INDIRA GANDHI (1917–1984)

Reviewing Alicia's activity monitoring in session revealed
important connections between her activities and mood. She had
never noticed a connection between her activities and her mood
before. The depression had just felt like something that loomed over
her, coloring everything. Worry and tension also seemed like constant
companions. She now recognized that there were many subtle shifts
in her mood, including some moments in which she experienced relief
from the depression and accompanying worry. She felt content when
she worked in her garden. After many weeks of avoiding friends, she
felt relief when she had dinner with her friend Ellen. It actually surprised her that Ellen was not angry with her and, in fact, expressed a
wish to be as supportive as possible.

As Alicia reviewed these activities with Beth, she also began to
identify activities that she could increase during the upcoming week
following their therapy session. Alicia thought that getting in touch
with more friends could be helpful for her mood. She told Beth that
she would call two friends from work, three old friends, and some
folks in her neighborhood. To her surprise, Beth asked her if she
thought that was too much to do right away. Beth explained that it

was often most helpful to work systematically and guarantee success by starting small. Alicia commented, "I thought I should force myself to do as much as possible now that we've figured out some things that might help." Beth explained: "It's terrific that we have some leads about what activities might help to boost your mood. My only caution is that planning too much between this session and next might leave you feeling demoralized if you don't accomplish it all. My hope is that we could develop a plan that is doable, one that won't feel overwhelming when you get started on it. What is one thing you feel pretty confident you could do this week in order to reconnect with some friends?" Alicia decided that seeing Ellen again for coffee would be the most logical place to start. If she could keep up that friendship, she reasoned, she would feel much better about herself. Plus, Ellen's social personality might benefit Alicia in helping her reconnect with old friends over time. She planned to set up a coffee date with Ellen either on Wednesday after work or on the following Saturday morning.

Alicia also enjoyed the contentment she usually felt when she worked in her pea patch. Beth asked what she might do the next week in her garden. Alicia realized that she needed to get some mulch, so they wrote down a plan for that activity as well. Beth gave Alicia a new activity schedule, and she began to write some of her plans for specific times in the coming week. On Saturday afternoon, she wrote that she would go to the nursery and purchase three bags of mulch. Since she knew that it would be quite likely that she'd buy the mulch and then let it sit in the bags, she also wrote "Spread the mulch in the garden" in the box for 11:00 A.M. on Sunday.

Beth asked her if she could think of anything that might get in the way of carrying out these plans. Alicia wondered if rainy weather might interfere; so, she wrote down "rain or shine" next to the time for spreading mulch. She and Beth agreed that she would report back to Beth about how she felt during these activities in the next session. She also was to continue monitoring her activities and mood during other times of the week.

Introduction

In this chapter, we get to the heart of behavioral activation, namely, scheduling and structuring activities. Once the therapist and client understand the baseline level of activity and have developed initial hypotheses about the function of the client's behavior, treatment moves directly to structuring and scheduling activities. As we've discussed previously, the behavioral model of depression posits that depression is the result of low levels of positive reinforcement and/or high levels of punishment. What, then, is the place of activation in behavioral treatment of depression? When people are depressed, especially when some of the symptoms that they exhibit include lethargy, withdrawal, and apathy, opportunities for behavior to be positively reinforced are diminished. Avoidance behaviors are very likely negatively reinforced such that the withdrawal behaviors will increase. The purpose of activating clients from a behavioral perspective is to increase the likelihood that they will come into contact with contingencies that will positively reinforce approach behaviors. In this chapter, we discuss core strategies in BA to facilitate activation.

How to Activate Clients

Most depressed people realize that increasing activity might well be helpful. In fact, many clients have told themselves on countless occasions, "Just get going!"—or they have been told to do so by others. The paradox of BA, thus, is that therapists are asking clients to do the very thing that clients have the most trouble doing. Withdrawal, lethargy, and loss of interest and pleasure are all symptoms of depression; so, how does a treatment designed to change these experiences work? This predicament, indeed, represents the promise and challenge of BA.

In Chapter 2 we presented 10 core principles of behavioral activation. Three of these—Principles 1, 4, and 5—relate specifically to activation and action plans. We discuss each below and how collectively they help BA therapists guide their clients to increase activation.

Principle 1: The key to changing how people feel is helping them change what they do.

As we have stated, negative moods create a momentum all of their own, and Principle 1 therefore encapsulates the main purpose of BA, namely, to get people to regulate their moods through their behavior. When one feels down, one is more likely to act in ways that keep moving in the direction of feeling down. Our friend and colleague Marsha Linehan often says, "Emotions love themselves." Feeling down tends to elicit actions that are consistent with feeling down. Most BA interventions ask clients to act according to a plan or goal rather than a feeling or an internal state. When we recommend activation interventions, we highlight the nature of negative moods and then ask clients to consider the possibility of acting from the "outside-in" rather than from the "inside-out" (Martell et al., 2001). A depressed client who does not derive pleasure from activities and feels tired and lethargic is less likely to engage in activities that he or she once enjoyed. The BA therapist turns this around and asks the client to act from the outside—that is, according to a goal or plan rather than according to a mood. The same depressed client, for example, would be asked to engage in some formerly enjoyed activity despite lack of interest or to increase activity in other ways on the principle that enjoyment would eventually return. The aim of "outside-in" action is to bring the client into contact with positive rewards in the environment and to reverse the negative momentum of depressed mood.

Some clients express concern that acting from the "outside-in" requires them to act "phony" or "fake." To a certain degree this is true. BA strategies do invite clients to act according to a plan rather than a feeling, which may feel unnatural or "fake." It can be helpful to think of the analogy of a right-handed person having a broken arm and needing to use her (or his) left hand for daily tasks. It would be awkward to use just one hand rather than both to get through the day, and it would be particularly awkward to rely exclusively on one's nondominant hand. The woman (or man) with the broken arm may even report that she feels that she is not herself when she is clumsily trying to make a cup of coffee or work on her computer with only her left hand. Such tasks would require more effort and commitment than they did before she broke her arm. Over time, however, she would become more proficient, and using her solo left hand would get easier. Broken arms heal, and she would eventually be able to use both hands and be "back to normal." This analogy aptly describes what we ask of our depressed clients. We ask them to engage in the clumsy, effortful, and perhaps unnatural feeling of doing activities to improve their mood from the "outside-in" until their depression begins to lift. Once they are feeling better, engagement in the routine activities of their daily lives feels more automatic and natural.

Another common "inside-out" concern that clients may express is that their depression is biological. These clients wonder if a behavioral approach can address the real problem if it is indeed something physiological. Many depressed clients are currently taking or have taken antidepressant medications with varying degrees of success. Others wonder whether starting antidepressant medication might be a better choice. The BA therapist can attest to the client that there are many ways to treat depression.

Both BA and cognitive therapy have been shown to be as effective as medication or nearly so in several randomized clinical trials (DeRubeis et al., 2005; Dimidjian et al., 2006). Cognitive and behavioral interventions also provide more enduring relapse prevention than medication alone (Hollon, Stewart, & Strunk, 2006). It may be helpful for clients to learn that therapy has long-term benefits that medications do not offer.

The BA therapist also may be assisted by being familiar with research studies that suggest that changing one's activity can have a direct impact on one's mood and biology. There is a large and growing literature on the use of exercise to improve depressive symptoms. Dunn, Trivedi, Kampert, Clark, and Chambliss (2005) demonstrated that participants who exercised according to the standards set by the American College of Sports Medicine over 3–5 days per week showed significantly greater decreases in depressive symptoms than a placebo group or groups that exercised at what they considered a "lower dose." Mather et al. (2002) demonstrated a moderate reduction in depressive symptoms for older adults diagnosed with major depressive disorder who participated in an exercise group activity and an improvement that was greater than that of individuals who participated in a socialization only group. Brown, Ford, Burton, Marshall, and Dobson (2005) found a relationship between increasing physical activity and a reduction in depressive symptoms in middle-aged women independent of preexisting physical or psychological health. These studies provide additional evidence that it is possible to change your mood by changing what you do.

Elliot Valenstein, Professor Emeritus of Psychology and Neuroscience at the University of Michigan, has noted that "there is no question that experiences (both prenatal and postnatal) shape brain anatomy and function and have a major impact on behavior and thought" (Valenstein, 1998, p. 141). Life experiences and activities have effects on physiological symptoms. Our behavior is biological, and our biology is influenced by our behavior. Following a 2004 expert workshop on "The Neurobiology of Exercise," a consensus paper by Dishman et al. (2006) helped expand research in the field of exercise neurobiology, concluding that "chronic physical activity improves brain health" (p. 346). These researchers also pointed out that animal studies have demonstrated that physical activity increases brain growth factors and may have neurogenerative influences and stimulate the development and growth of new cells, protecting against ischemic neuronal damage in the hippocampal formation and nerotoxic damage in the neostriatum (Dishman et al., 2006, p. 346).

Clinical research with humans also has indicated that changes in brain chemistry can be achieved without medical or pharmacological intervention. Schwartz, Stoessel, Baxter, Martin, and Phelps (1996) found that participants diagnosed with obsessive–compulsive disorder (OCD) who responded to behavior therapy had significantly greater changes in an area of the brain associated with glucose metabolic activity after treatment than those who did not respond to behavior therapy. Although this study was limited by a very small sample size (9 participants), a larger study with 22 participants also demonstrated significant decreases in regional cerebral blood flow in this area following successful behavior therapy for OCD (Nakatani et al., 2003). Research on the neural mechanisms involved following response to CBT treatment of other problems, like social phobia, have shown similar results (Furmark et al., 2003).

Neuroimaging studies of depressed clients successfully treated with CBT have also been conducted. Reciprocal limbic increases and cortical decreases were identified through neuroimaging following successful treatment with CBT (Goldapple et al., 2004). The authors of these studies speculate that the metabolic change pattern that is seen following successful CBT treatment may provide neural correlates of the proposed psychological mechanisms that mediate a response to CBT such as directed attention, reward-based decision making, monitoring of emotional salience, memory function, self-referential processing, and cognitive ruminations. A multisite meta-analysis of brain imaging scans at baseline involving brain regions associated with depression identified in previous studies has also shown differing patterns of neural activation between medication responders and CBT responders (Seminowicz et al., 2004). Although the specific pattern of change in neural activation over the course of treatment was different for patients receiving medication in comparison with patients receiving psychosocial treatment, the successful implementation of each treatment modality was associated with significant changes in brain activity. Numerous studies have shown the effects of cognitive therapy to be enduring, whereas the effects of antidepressant medications do not reduce the future risk of relapse (DeRubeis, Siegle, & Hollon, 2008). While there are as yet no data on neuroimaging following treatment with BA, studies conducted with cognitive therapy or CBT support the assertion that nonpharmacological interventions can produce observable biological changes. Acute treatment response to BA was shown to be superior to that of cognitive therapy, and long-term survival rates (followed for 2 years) for those successfully treated with BA were not significantly different from CT in a large randomized clinical trial. Significantly more participants who had responded to prior antidepressant medication (paroxetine) relapsed when the medication was discontinued than participants who had responded to 24 sessions or fewer of prior CT or prior BA (Dimidjian et al., 2006; Dobson et al., 2008). While we have no observations of brain activity for clients successfully treated with BA, we can speculate that the behavior change targeted in BA may have a similar impact on neural activity as that of CBT. BA clients are encouraged to increase a variety of activities, from engaging in the complex process of work or family demands to simple exercise. Clients are encouraged to take an overall active stance, to participate in productive problem solving rather than ruminate over problems, and to engage in behaviors that are opposite to avoidance.

Consistent daily activation has been shown to be a protective factor for both mental and physical health. Leisure activities in particular have been shown to lead to well-being in adolescents, adults, and the elderly by increasing coping abilities in the face of life stressors, including daily hassles (Caldwell, 2005). Chung (2004) found that elderly residents in nursing homes in Hong Kong who were able to engage in activities of daily living and leisure had a greater sense of well-being than those who did not engage in such activities.

There is also increasing evidence that meaningful work has an important impact on mental health. Mallinckrodt and Bennet (1992) found that recently unemployed blue-collar workers were more depressed than those who remained consistently employed, although social support was a protective factor for those who had been laid off from their jobs. Blustein (2008) states that "working is a central ingredient in the development and sustenance of psychological health" (p. 230). It is important to remember that daily meaningful work is a source of satisfaction and well-being. On the other hand, simply finding another job does not necessarily enable people who have lost a job to return to baseline levels of life satisfaction (Lucas, Clark, Georgellis, & Diener, 2004). This finding is consistent with our view that BA therapists do not offer simple solutions to clients' problems, and therefore "just getting a new job" would never be considered a sufficient treatment for depression. Nevertheless, most of many adults' social networks, as well as their sense of accomplishment, will be found in their workplace or through professional connections.

It may be helpful for therapists to refer to this knowledge base when inviting a client to try BA strategies. Clients may be encouraged by knowing that there are multiple lines of scientific research that support the basic model that activation can improve mood. Armed with such information, therapists and clients can begin the task of deciding which activities are most appropriate to focus on and in what forms to begin the work from the "outside-in."

Principle 4: Structure and schedule activities that follow a plan, not a mood.

The behavioral assessment process helps the therapist and the client select an activity and develop a solid rationale for why it is an important activity to target. The next step is to schedule and structure the activity. The rationale for scheduling activities is that identifying a specific time (and sometimes, place) for an activity will help to maximize activation. Not all activation assignments will involve scheduling; for instance, a client may leave a session with a general agreement to call a friend prior to the next session. However, specifically scheduling an activity can be often very helpful since many clients have good intentions to do things but are subject to mood-dependent behaviors that get in the way of accomplishing plans. Scheduling refers to setting a particular time when the client will commit to doing that activity and provides a convenient anchor for clients to act upon rather than seeing how they feel at the time. If appropriate, the therapist and client also agree upon the duration of the activity. Structuring the activity involves defining what the client will do in behavioral terms, deciding where the activity will occur, whether other people will be involved, and how the client will measure success.

Decide How Frequently the Task Should Occur

As we have discussed previously, clients often overestimate what can be achieved early on. Deciding the frequency of occurrence for a particular task needs to follow the principle of starting small and gradually building up the iterations. Take, for example, a client who states that he would like to start jogging again and plans to do so every day prior to the next session. Although such frequency might have been easy to accomplish when he was running regularly prior to getting depressed, it is likely to be challenging at this time. BA therapists aim to guide clients to start with a frequency that evokes confidence from both the client and therapist. The therapist may suggest that the client take one run per week. The client may not want to schedule jogging only one time during the week and may wish to run three times. As a start, this might be fine, and the client can always do more if he is able. The next important step is to decide the intensity and duration of the activity.

Decide the Duration and/or Intensity of the Activity

Consider a similar situation with James, a client who leaves a session early in therapy with the assignment to take a walk once each day for 3 days prior to his next appointment. What might be a limitation of this assignment? Certainly, it appears a promising approach for getting the client physically active, and it is clear how many times the activity will occur. However, the assignment may lack specificity that could guide James in a helpful way. One question a therapist can reflect on is, Does this assignment give us both enough information so that the agreement we are making is clear? In BA, a high value is placed on behavioral specificity. Is James agreeing to walk for 2 hours, 10 minutes, or perhaps 3 miles 3 days per week? If it used to take James 45 minutes to walk 3 miles, it might be a good idea for him to set the maximum duration at 20 minutes three times a week for the first week.

Decide on the Specific Days and Times That the Client Will Do the Activity

With repeated review of a client's activity charts, the therapist begins to develop a clear picture of the current range of activities. In this context, the therapist and the client need to identify days and times that will maximize the likelihood that the activity will be completed. James, who agreed to walk 3 days a week, reveals that he is most likely to walk first thing in the morning when he hasn't lost momentum as the day unfolds. First the therapist considers when he needs to be at work, how early he would need to leave his house to go walking, and whether it is feasible to walk first thing in the morning. A client who is barely getting up in time to make it to work is not likely to be able to jump out of bed an hour earlier to complete a 20-minute walk. James can then decide which days may be better for his work schedule. James can then write "walk for 20 minutes" in his activity monitoring chart (see Figure 5.1) on the specific days and times agreed upon.

Principle 5: Change will be easier when starting small.

This simple idea is a critical part of helping clients effectively activate. We can make a cake from a recipe by measuring out each of the ingredients, mixing the dry and then the wet ingredients, and then combining them, but we don't make a cake by throwing all of the ingredients at once into a greased pan, stirring, and tossing it into the oven. Similarly, activities need to be broken down into behaviorally specific definable parts, particularly when one is coping with depression.

Unfortunately, many of us often forget these simple truths. One may anticipate reconnecting with old friends as well as family on a week-long trip back to a childhood home, only to find that there is not enough time to see even half of the people as planned. Early on a sunny Saturday morning, it might seem that one can get all of the yard work done, only to find that dinnertime arrives and more of the

	Mon.	Tues.	Wed.	Thurs.	Fri.	Sat.	Sun.
5:00 A.M.–7:00 A.M.		*Walk for 20 minutes*					
8:00 A.M.	*8:30 Leave for work*	*8:30 Leave for work*	*8:30 Leave for work*	*8:30 Leave for work*	*8:30 Leave for work*		
9:00 A.M.							
10:00 A.M.							
11:00 A.M.						*Walk for 20 minutes*	
12:00 P.M.							
1:00 P.M.							
2:00 P.M.							*Walk for 20 minutes*
3:00 P.M.							
4:00 P.M.							
5:00 P.M.							
6:00 P.M.							
7:00 P.M.							
8:00 P.M.							
9:00 P.M.							
10:00 P.M.							
11:00 P.M.–5:00 A.M.							
12:00 A.M.							

FIGURE 5.1. James's activity monitoring chart.

job remains. Such patterns are common, but they are also particularly difficult when one is depressed. BA offers an alternative, namely, graded task assignment.

Encouraged throughout treatment, graded task assignment involves working with clients to start small and build from there. A graded task is one that starts with the simplest components and builds in complexity and difficulty; thus, assigning activities occurs in a stepwise fashion, moving from simple to more complex. Designing assignments in this way sets up the likelihood that there will be early success when the client attempts the activity. The reason for this is to ensure that treatment is experienced as rewarding, not punishing for failing to complete early steps that may be too difficult. Allowing the idea that activity breeds activity, early success can result in a sense of accomplishment that can foster motivation to undertake future assignments.

Locke and Latham (1990) observed that performance is enhanced when people set themselves challenging but specific goals rather than challenging but vague goals. Moreover, immediate goals are associated with better performance than are long-term goals (Bandura & Schunk, 1981). Intentions about how goals will be implemented, which specify the when, where, and how of action, are also critical elements of goal attainment (Gollwitzer, 1999; Gollwitzer & Brandstätter, 1997). Promotion goals, which focus on the presence or absence of positive outcomes, also appear to have advantages in facilitating action as compared to prevention goals, which focus on the presence or absence of negative outcomes. These findings can help to inform the activity structuring efforts of the therapist and client.

Above all else, the place to start grading tasks is with baseline data. It is necessary to begin where the client currently is functioning, not where the client believes he or she should be functioning. When a client has been coping with depression for a long while, making changes is likely to take time.

When Alicia committed to getting in touch with friends, Beth needed to remember to start small and to keep breaking the task down as much as possible.

BETH: So, we've talked about your need to get connected with friends.

ALICIA: Yes, I can't just keep avoiding everyone. I'll really be utterly alone.

BETH: What happens when you think about calling friends?

ALICIA: In the morning, I just roll over and stay in bed. I just feel so tired and down. It's all just too hard. In the evening, I find anything to do but call.

BETH: Have you made any steps toward calling or seeing friends?

ALICIA: No, none, not since getting together with Ellen. There are so many people it seems, but I'm feeling overwhelmed by all of it. I think I should meet this woman from work who seems nice and wants to get to know me. I haven't talked with Bobby in about 5 months, and he had said he wanted to get together before last Christmas! I guess I need to see Bobby.

BETH: Doing all of that sounds like a lot, Alicia.

ALICIA: ... and there are my sister and brother—when I think about it all I want to just crawl into a hole.

BETH: I understand. It is overwhelming to look at dealing with everyone all at once. Getting reconnected with your friends is a big task. You've made several smaller steps, however, like meeting with Ellen that one time. I wonder about some more small steps you could take. What do you think about making a list of some of the specific activities that are involved in rebuilding the social connections in your life? Then, we can see what might be a helpful place to start.

ALICIA: Okay.

BETH: It sounds like you already have the list of people in your life with whom you could reach out in some ways. What if we ranked those in terms of who was easiest and who was hardest?

ALICIA: That's easy. My brother and then sister are at the top, then probably Bobby because I've put it off for so long, and then the person at work. Probably Ellen would be the easiest. I guess I could start there.

BETH: That makes sense to me. I also like that idea because it seems like reconnecting with Ellen might have the highest odds of having a positive impact on your mood now. Is that right?

ALICIA: Yes, she's been pretty supportive.

BETH: What do you think would happen if you started by setting a goal for yourself of getting together with Ellen again once this coming week?

ALICIA: I don't know …

BETH: Sounds like something might get in the way.

ALICIA: I think it would be a big production.

BETH: Yes, that's a good observation. Sounds like we could break down the task more! What about starting with something like asking her to grab a cup of coffee with you on one afternoon?

ALICIA: I guess I could do that.

BETH: When would you do that?

ALICIA: Maybe tomorrow. I usually feel a little more motivated after our sessions.

BETH: What if you wake up feeling absolutely unmotivated?

ALICIA: I don't know. That is pretty typical.

BETH: One option would be to remind yourself of what we have talked about with "outside-in" and "inside-out" activities—do you think that might help? We could even make a reminder sign now that you could post somewhere where you could see it when you wake up.

ALICIA: That might help me.

BETH: The other option is that you actually call her today, right after our session.

ALICIA: That's true. That might be better. I could at least call and see if she is available for tomorrow.

BETH: I think the key here is finding a place to begin. I know this is really hard. It's been a stressful issue for a long time, and it may take a bit of effort to solve this problem. I'm very confident we can figure this out, though. I'm going to ask you to not expect more of yourself than having one cup of coffee with Ellen this week.

ALICIA: Okay, I can do that, provided she is available.

BETH: Let's write down making the call for today after our session and then perhaps block your schedule for several days to make sure you hit on a day when she's available.

ALICIA: I guess that is the best way to make sure I actually do it.

BETH: Let's talk about where you might have coffee that will make this doable ...

In this exchange Beth works with Alicia to break down the task of social engagement. On occasion, clients who are having considerable trouble with simple tasks actually get a lot more accomplished once they start. Alicia may find that she starts with a call to Ellen and then follows with reconnecting with her friend Bobby later in the week. Breaking tasks down requires creativity on the part of the therapist and client. Some tasks are relatively straightforward, such as cleaning a room or paying overdue bills. Other tasks, such as building interpersonal connections or grieving an important loss, can be quite complex. Regardless of the task complexity, however, the intention is to get the client started on something. It is clear that simply meeting with one friend is not likely to alleviate depression. Yet, the BA therapist returns again and again to the principle of "start small and build from there." Changing little things can bring a sense of accomplishment and a glimmer of hope, increasing the likelihood that clients will continue to reengage in ever more difficult and important elements of their lives. This can be particularly important when tackling problems that are complicated by not only the client's depression but also the nature of the context of their lives. For example, jobs can be difficult to find, and the process of job seeking can maintain and increase depression over time.

John had been laid off from his job as a salesman many months ago. It had been his dream to start his own business and be his own boss. He thought he could cope with the vicissitudes of the economy and did not want to put himself at the mercy of another company. After a few months of efforts to launch a business, however, he found himself frustrated and feeling down. When he sought therapy, he was stuck. He spent most days at home and explained to his therapist that he couldn't even say what he did all day. He still had some hope for his own business, but he was clearly caught in the trap of not knowing where to begin. Fortunately, John had received a small severance payment from his job, and his wife was working full-time; so, there was enough money for him to spend some time figuring this out. The problem was that time was ticking by and he was not moving forward.

With the help of his therapist, John started to think small. The first step was to look around at the types of jobs people had that allowed them to be independent, work outdoors, and move around during the day. As an initial assignment, he explored landscaping, yard work, staging yards and homes for realtors, dog walking, and painting houses. He and his therapist discussed what he learned about each possible option. Of these ideas, doing something with animals particularly appealed to him. He thought that it would take very little training to learn to manage dogs, and so he decided to explore the possibility of opening a dog walking and exercising business. He had taken the first small step of making a decision about the kind of business he might like to pursue.

With his therapist's guidance, John began to build his job concept with a series of small steps. First, he evaluated the market in his local area for such a business. He also attended several dog-training classes with his own dog so that he'd be able to offer some level of obedience training as part of a package for his customers. He next got the proper business license and joined an association of professional pet sitters. He then developed brochures and a marketing plan.

After 6 months he had his first three customers. He wasn't making enough money to support himself, but he was moving forward. His mood had steadily improved with each step of the task. While he was still a bit worried about finances, he actually felt joy when working with the dogs.

In summary, starting small is a big part of BA! It counters the tendency to set ineffectual goals and helps clients move forward in productive ways. Setting goals that feel overwhelming is particularly common when people are depressed. Many clients will argue that doing a few steps is not enough and that they should do more. At the opposite end of the "can do" continuum, some clients will say "I can't do it" to even the smallest of tasks. Emphasizing the need to start small can often provide relief on both ends of the spectrum. Setting out detailed graded task assignments can be extremely helpful when one is depressed.

In all of these ways, the BA therapist balances the client's need to change against the realities of the client's energy, time, and resources. The process of change using graded tasks often requires patience and perseverance on the part of both the client and therapist. Table 5.1 provides two additional examples of ways in which therapists and cli-

TABLE 5.1. Two Examples of Grading Complex Tasks

Reengaging with friends.
- Make a list of people with whom the client has lost contact.
- Gather as many current telephone numbers or e-mail addresses as possible for those individuals.
- Choose one or two people to contact.
- Choose a day, time, and method for contacting them.
- Make the call or send the e-mail.
- Invite the person to meet face-to-face.
- Identify another old friend.
- Repeat.

Improving an unsatisfying work context in which a client feels overwhelmed and is falling behind on important work projects.
- List all the work projects.
- Record the deadline for each project or indicate if projects are ongoing.
- Identify one project to target in the coming week.
- Identify the specific subcomponents of that project.
- Record the amount of time estimated for each subcomponent.
- Schedule one subcomponent task each morning.
- Monitor the amount of time spent, what was accomplished, and the barriers that arose.
- Bring the monitoring form back to the next session to troubleshoot and choose a new project for the next target.

Note. Some activities are easier to grade than others. Relationship- and employment-related goals can be complicated. Illustrated here are some ways in which a therapist and client graded such tasks.

From *Behavioral Activation for Depression: A Clinician's Guide* by Christopher R. Martell, Sona Dimidjian, and Ruth Herman-Dunn. Copyright 2010 by The Guilford Press. Permission to photocopy this table is granted to purchasers of this book for personal use only (see copyright page for details). Purchasers may download a larger version of this table from the book's page on The Guilford Press website.

ents have broken down activities to make changes in some important life domains.

Countering All-or-Nothing Activation

Activity scheduling and structuring can counter client avoidance and help clients begin activating. The goal, however, is not necessarily to complete a task in its entirety. Many depressed clients easily succumb to a sense of failure and set goals that are unrealistic. Activities should be set up to maximize success. For example, if an agreed-upon assignment was to call or visit two specific friends over the course of the week, talking to one friend even one time on the telephone is viewed as a success upon which to build. Sometimes an activity provides an immediate boost in mood, making it easier to reattempt the process (as in the earlier example when Ellen told Alicia how happy she was to hear from her). At other times encouragement to continue is needed, and therapists can reassure clients that, while not immediately rewarding, a correctly chosen activity should eventually become so. This is frequently the case when activities involve chores such as cleaning a room, writing a résumé, and the like. A client may or may not feel happy as a result of no longer having leaves cluttering his yard, and a client might complete the task even without feeling good being outdoors. Nevertheless, making ongoing incremental attempts at yard work may be experienced as pleasurable over time. Additionally, BA is as much about engaging in mastery activities as pleasure, and we cannot underestimate the reinforcement value of mastery. For example, although the client may not have enjoyed the yard work, he may have felt satisfaction at completing the task. Even small steps can be rewarding, though the reward may not be readily apparent. BA is based on the premise that if clients continue to take small steps over time they will eventually get back on track.

Principle 6: Emphasize activities that are naturally reinforcing.

When people engage in behavior that is reinforced naturally in the environment, it has a greater likelihood of reoccurrence than does behavior that is reinforced arbitrarily by adding something externally that is not necessarily related to the behavior—such as giving a child candy to reward taking a bath. Natural reinforcement means that reinforcing consequences follow logically from the behavior and are indigenous to the environment (Sulzer-Azaroff & Mayr, 1991). For example, if an individual cleans dishes because it provides a sense of accomplishment and enjoyment when seeing the kitchen looking tidy, dishwashing behavior is likely to increase. The sense of mastery and pleasure are natural contingencies, following logically from the act of washing dishes. In contrast, if a person experiences washing dishes only as a chore and finds the entire experience aversive but receives a treat after finishing, the dishes might get washed once or twice, but the specific behavior of dishwashing will not necessarily be permanently increased.

If Alicia's friend Ellen responded to a call by saying "It is about time you called—I thought you'd dropped off the Earth!," Alicia might feel ashamed and saddened by her telephone conversation with Ellen. However if Ellen were to respond with "Alicia, it is so great to hear from you, I've been thinking of you and wanting to call you myself—glad you beat me to it!," Alicia would likely feel accepted, happy, and be more inclined to call again. These are natural contingencies, and Ellen's approval might serve as a natural reinforcer.

Thus, the skillful BA therapist works to identify activities that have a high likelihood of natural reinforcement. The clues to activities that are naturally reinforcing lie in the client's history of what has occurred in the past. The simple question "What are you likely to do when you're not depressed?" may help to uncover such activities.

Managing the contingencies in clients' lives is one way to make good use of natural reinforcement. Contingency management means simply managing the outcome of activities under certain circumstances, that is, managing the "ABCs" of behavior. For example, a therapist can encourage a client to make a public commitment to engage in a certain activity. James, the client discussed earlier who agreed to walk for 20 minutes three times over the next week can be encouraged to experiment with taking a walk with a friend rather than alone. Agreeing to walk with a friend is a type of public commitment that may also increase the sense of pleasure that follows naturally from sharing an activity with someone else. On some occasions the therapist and client may agree on a plan that the client will call the therapist when a task is completed. This serves two possible purposes: The behavior may be reinforced by the sense of accomplishment the client feels in telling the therapist about a success, and avoidance may be reduced because the client doesn't want to admit to the therapist that the task wasn't completed.

Another method of contingency management is to use the Premack (1959) principle that restricts engaging in a high-frequency behavior subject to first engaging in a low-frequency behavior. In other words, if watching television is a high-frequency behavior and cleaning the kitchen is a low-frequency behavior, one could make watching television contingent on first spending a specified amount of time cleaning the kitchen. This approach accords with the principle of engaging in behaviors that are naturally reinforcing, but it uses other inducements to increase engagement in behaviors that are less reinforcing. Admittedly, it utilizes a reinforcing activity arbitrarily since, in our example, watching television is not a natural result of cleaning a kitchen. Nevertheless, tedious or difficult tasks can also be made easier by managing environmental contingencies. Listening to music while cleaning may make cleaning more enjoyable. Grading tasks in order to start with one that can be accomplished quickly may give an immediate sense of mastery and increase motivation to tackle a more time-consuming or difficult task. Managing contingencies, scheduling activities, and setting behavioral goals that are attainable for the client are consistent techniques used throughout BA.

TABLE 5.2. Structuring and Scheduling Activities for BA

When helping clients to structure and schedule activities, often it is helpful to keep the following considerations in mind:

- What task frequency will be most effectual for the client?
- What duration and/or intensity of the activity will be most effectual for the client?
- On what specific days and at what times should the client do the activity?
- Have you and the client started "small"?
- Have you and the client countered "all-or-nothing activation"?
- Have you and the client identified activities that are likely to be naturally reinforcing?

From *Behavioral Activation for Depression: A Clinician's Guide* by Christopher R. Martell, Sona Dimidjian, and Ruth Herman-Dunn. Copyright 2010 by The Guilford Press. Permission to photocopy this table is granted to purchasers of this book for personal use only (see copyright page for details). Purchasers may download a larger version of this table from the book's page on The Guilford Press website.

Summary

We have stressed the importance of scheduling and structuring activities so that clients are more likely to increase activation. Table 5.2 provides a summary of ideas for working with this technique. In order to help depressed clients to engage in antidepressant behaviors, BA therapists and clients work together to schedule specific activities for clients to complete between sessions. Each activity is structured in advance so that clients know specifically what they have agreed to do. Activities should be consistent with clients' long- or short-term goals. There are clues to be found in a client's history about past activities that he or she has found engaging, which may naturally reinforce the client's antidepressant behaviors. Potential problems that might get in the way of activation are discussed in advance, with a particular emphasis on possible avoidance behaviors. We now turn to a more thorough discussion of problem solving and specific ways to counter avoidance behaviors.

6

Solving Problems
and Countering Avoidance

There are risks and costs to a program of action. But they are
far less than the long-range risks and costs of comfortable
inaction.
—JOHN F. KENNEDY (1917–1963)

Alicia told her therapist: "My life is such a mess, and I'm so far
from where I want to be. My friendships are in shambles, and I feel
miserable about it. Sometimes I just wonder, what's the point?"

Beth listened carefully to Alicia talk about the difficulties in the
interpersonal domain of her life and the ways in which such problems
were connected to her ongoing depression. Alicia explained: "The
only person who even calls me anymore is Ellen. Why would anyone
else want to when I haven't been returning their calls and they have
to go to such an ugly part of town to see me? It's all I can do to get up
to go to my temp job—and in fact, that's pretty much all I'm doing—
but it's no way to live."

Beth understood the magnitude of the challenges that were facing Alicia. She communicated this to her and then asked specifically
about the problems with her job. She said: "I agree, Alicia. It sounds
like you have very little that's meaningful or fun in your life right
now, and you're spending an awful lot of time in an environment that
you don't like. I know we've been starting to work on your friendships, and I'm wondering too about the ways in which your work
situation is impacting your mood. Have you sidelined your goal of
finding better employment?"

Alicia's response was clear. "What's the point? I looked for 8 months just to get this silly temp job; so, yes, I guess so. I've kind of given up on a lot of things. It seems like all I have the energy or motivation for is to lie in bed and thumb through stupid magazines. Why can't I just get myself to go job hunting again or pick up the phone and call my friends?"

Beth commented in return: "Alicia, this sounds like something we talked about when we first met. It's that kind of just force yourself to Just do it! approach through willpower that doesn't work very well with depression. Taking action and solving life's problems is hard, Alicia, especially when you're feeling depressed. Remember that it's for these reasons that having a coach like me to help you figure all this out can be particularly helpful. Together, we will determine specifically what the problems are that keep you stuck and from moving ahead in your life. I'm wondering which area is a better place for us to start working on—friends or work?" Alicia replied: "The job thing is too hard right now. I don't think I can do that when I am feeling like this. Plus, I think if I had some more support it might be easier to do the job stuff." "I agree completely." said Beth, "Let's pick up there again today."

Introduction

Alicia began her session with a strong sense of hopelessness, asking directly, "What's the point?" Many therapists have heard a similar lament from their depressed clients. The clients feel overwhelmed by the sheer number and difficulty of their problems, and at times it is easy for the therapist to become overwhelmed as well. Often clients are depressed because they have real-world problems and find themselves in extraordinarily difficult and painful situations. Some clients also begin therapy with coping strategies characterized by passivity, avoidance, or withdrawal. As discussed, these coping responses create additional secondary problems that can maintain depression over time. Many clients feel as though they are caught in a totally darkened cave and cannot find their way out into the sunlight.

Solving problems effectively is one pathway out of depression. Given the emphasis in BA on contextual factors that maintain depression over time, solving problems takes a front-and-center role, occurring throughout the course of therapy. The job of the BA therapist is to "Act as a coach" (Principle 7), and much of this coaching focuses on helping the client to solve problems. As Principle 8 states, "Emphasize a problem-solving empirical approach, and recognize that all results are useful." This principle is a constant thread throughout all BA sessions, as therapists engage with clients in solving important life problems and as therapists embody a problem-solving stance in their reactions to problems that may arise over the course of treatment. In this chapter we discuss the ways in which solving problems is accomplished in BA. We provide an overview of traditional problem-solving interventions as a foundation from which to discuss how therapists approach problems in BA. We also provide an acronym that serves as a helpful mnemonic when conducting problem solving in BA.

Traditional Problem Solving and Its Use in BA

Problem solving is a tried-and-true cognitive-behavioral technique that is utilized in BA and has been extensively studied as a treatment in its own right (D'Zurilla & Nezu, 1999; Mynors-Wallis et al., 1997). Traditional problem solving has a long history; it has been applied to a variety of target problems and populations, including both individuals (D'Zurilla & Goldfried, 1971; D'Zurilla & Nezu, 1982) and couples (Jacobson & Margolin, 1979).

Traditional problem solving typically proceeds in a structured fashion. Consistent with our recommendation that BA therapists be specific and concrete, the first step is to define the problem clearly. Carefully defining problems can help address clients' feeling overwhelmed by the magnitude of their problems. Problems are defined in behavioral terms so that it is easier to generate solutions. One can imagine several solutions to a problem such as "I spend too much time staring into space, thinking about how much I miss my best friend, who moved." In contrast, it is more difficult to generate solutions to a problem defined simply as "I feel badly." It is helpful to guide clients in developing the habit of stating problems in behavioral terms and thinking contextually about the situations in which the problems occur.

The second step in problem solving is to brainstorm as many solutions as possible without judging them. Not judging possible solutions allows one to generate diverse possibilities rather than stick to just a few practical solutions. Once a broad list of possibilities is generated, they can be evaluated in terms of the pros and cons of each solution. The client and therapist may spend a good deal of time on this step. Discussing the pros and cons of solutions from a list of possible options helps to clarify the best course of action. Once the client has decided on a particular solution, it should be stated in behavioral terms and put into practice.

The next step in the process is to evaluate the outcome. In order to do this, a realistic time frame for experimenting with a solution is necessary. Once the client has implemented the solution over the predetermined course of time, the outcome of the solution can be assessed. At this point it may be necessary to modify the solution or generate a different solution altogether.

Problem solving in BA is not necessarily taught using these specific steps in an explicit or didactic manner. In some ways, the emphasis in BA is on "solving problems" rather than explicitly "teaching problem solving." Therapists work actively with clients to identify problems that are triggering or maintaining depression and to solve them. In so doing, the BA therapist asks questions to define the problem, generates solutions, and assesses the outcome of plans that are developed.

For example, one client, Timothy, wanted to purchase a new car because his current car got poor gas mileage and required expensive repairs. His partner, Gail, had expressed concern about how much money they spent, and Timothy was worried about disapproval at home. He and his therapist had the following exchange:

TIMOTHY: I want to get a car, but I'm sure Gail is going to be angry if I ask her.

THERAPIST: Have the two of you talked about getting a new car?

TIMOTHY: No. She got really angry with me last month when I came home with a new flat-screen television that one of my office colleagues was selling for only $300!

THERAPIST: Had you talked about getting a new television?

TIMOTHY: We'd said we might buy ourselves a flat-screen television for Christmas next year. I thought this was a great deal, and I couldn't believe how angry she got when I brought it home.

THERAPIST: Had she gotten angry about spending the money?

TIMOTHY: Well, I think it was the fact that I didn't ask her before I bought it. She enjoys watching it now, though.

THERAPIST: So, she got angry because you didn't consult her before buying the television from your friend. Is there anything to learn from that in terms of how to address the new car dilemma?

TIMOTHY: Well, I guess I shouldn't just go out and buy one without talking to her about it first.

THERAPIST: That sounds reasonable. How might you address this—what are some possibilities?

TIMOTHY: Well, I could just go get one, but, like I said, that's probably a bad idea. I suppose I could tell her I really think my current car is costing us a whole lot of money in the long run and that it would be cheaper to get a new car.

THERAPIST: How would you make that claim?

TIMOTHY: Oh, that's easy. I have receipts from the last 3 months alone of repair bills. $3,200! I also have kept a watch on mileage, and my car is getting only 22 miles to the gallon! I think a hybrid would be a better deal.

THERAPIST: So, you could present that data to her. Anything else you might do?

TIMOTHY: I could probably go online and look up the price of newer, but not brand-new, hybrids and see the mileage ratings.

THERAPIST: Yes. So, what would you accomplish by all of this?

TIMOTHY: I'd be giving her a good rationale and showing her that this isn't just an impulse buy.

THERAPIST: Is that important to her?

TIMOTHY: I think so. I mean she really was mad that I didn't call her before buying the TV, although she did agree that the price was right. So, I think I should gather this information and talk with her about this.

THERAPIST: When will you do this?

TIMOTHY: I have all the receipts, and I could go online tomorrow. Maybe I should get it over with and talk with her tomorrow night.

THERAPIST: Shall we put that on your activity schedule?

TIMOTHY: Sure.

THERAPIST: Is there anything else you would do?

TIMOTHY: Maybe ask her if she'd like to take a day next weekend and just look at cars. Maybe just have some fun test-driving. I'd even promise not to buy anything right away that weekend.

THERAPIST: It sounds like a very workable plan to me. I'm wondering how we can evaluate its success. How will we know that this solution to this problem has worked?

TIMOTHY: I'd get a car.

THERAPIST: So, if she doesn't agree that you can buy a car, you will have failed?

TIMOTHY: Well, I guess that's pretty severe. Maybe I'd feel like this was a success if we actually talked about this without getting into an argument.

THERAPIST: Do you think your plan is sufficient to try to guarantee that?

TIMOTHY: If I also tell her upfront that I just want to talk about this—because I do respect her opinion and input—and that I'm not demanding that she see things my way.

THERAPIST: That all sounds like a reasonable plan to try. Let's talk next week about how it all works out.

In this exchange the therapist helps Timothy to identify the problem that had occurred with buying the new television. It was not, in fact, the purchase but rather the lack of consultation with his partner that got her upset, which clarified the nature of the problem to be solved when discussing Timothy's desire to get a new car. Timothy also generated solutions that might not work as well and those that would possibly work better. Once he had a plan, he scheduled a time to implement it. Knowing that it might be unrealistic to anticipate that his partner would simply agree as a result of the plan, the therapist asked Timothy for more specificity about determining success.

Types of Problems Addressed in BA

There are two general categories of problems that BA targets: primary and secondary problems. Primary problems, which are normally beyond the client's control, influence both the initiation and maintenance of depression, while secondary problems result from the client's natural response to the primary problems. For example, primary problems might include having a history of family instability or the current break-up of a relationship. A particular individual's reaction to these might be to feel hopeless and lethargic, and, if serious enough, these symptoms would be diagnosed as depression. Staying in bed, avoiding friends, or participating in passive activities (like watching television) are understandable responses when one feels lethargic. Keeping a low social profile is also reasonable when one has been hurt or when interpersonal difficulties stir up negative emotions from one's adverse family history. BA considers such behaviors secondary problems since they serve to maintain the depressed mood and can exacerbate the primary problem—in this case, keeping the person ultimately more isolated and alone because of the loss of contact with friends as well as because of the loss of the relationship. Although secondary problems may be exacerbated by client skill deficits, they are typically under greater control by the client and therefore may initially be more amenable to intervention.

Primary problems may include experiences of loss that have made life less rewarding and/or more punishing, daily hassles, and such negative events as an injury that creates chronic pain or a series of small changes such as a new neighbor that adds noise pollution or an increase in traffic. Secondary problems can consist of social withdrawal, passive escapist behaviors like playing computer games, or the abuse of alcohol or drugs. Another way to say this is that primary problems represent an event or events that may well trigger depression, while secondary problems occur as a result of common but ineffectual responses to feeling depressed.

Although primary problems are important targets for change, they are often targeted after some progress has been made on secondary problems. Primary problems can be more difficult to solve when one is depressed. Secondary problems, on the other hand, are easier to target once it becomes clear what is being avoided and what function this avoidance serves. Since the tendency to escape or avoid negative feelings and situations is very human, addressing primary problems before helping clients develop the ability to activate in the face of negative feelings may result in limited success and leave clients feeling even more discouraged. Once the client has started to increase activation, it can be easier to tackle primary problems.

Keep in mind that whether a problem is primary or secondary cannot always be determined from the behavior's form; rather, attending to the function of the problem behavior often is necessary. For example, losing a job can be a primary problem that precipitates a depressive episode and is completely beyond the control of the client due to a declining economy. Conversely, losing a job could be the result of a behavioral pattern for someone who, in response to feeling depressed, shows up late or not at all and is consequently fired. This is a clear example of how in one instance the job loss is independent of the person's behavior and is thus a primary problem while in the other case it is a direct consequence of avoidance and is thus a secondary problem.

Problem Solving and Avoidance

As avoidance is one of the most frequent barriers to effective problem solving, countering client avoidance is a critical part of solving problems in BA. Two elements are critical in this process, namely identifying when avoidance is occurring and validating the client's dilemma. We first address how to identify avoidance and then turn our attention to the importance of validating the difficulty of changing avoidance patterns.

Therapists can identify avoidance by being on the alert for behavior that helps a client keep something aversive from happening. We also use the general term "avoidance" as a shortcut when talking to clients about both avoidance behaviors—that is, acting in order to prevent something—and escape behaviors—that is, taking oneself out of an undesirable situation—when clients do something to temporarily escape from an aversive experience. Unhelpful escape behaviors include turning on the television to escape from having to prepare tax documents, drinking alcohol to escape from feelings of loneliness, and so forth. To the extent that the behavior is more likely to recur as a result of such escape and avoidance, we can then say that it has been negatively reinforced. In addition, while the client may receive short-term benefit from the avoidance behavior, there is almost always a cost. Typically, the client is not approaching some activity that is required to pursue important long-term goals and well-being. This, in a nutshell, describes the way avoidance is conceptualized in BA. Avoidance is at times obvious—for example, when clients isolate themselves in their apartment all weekend, neglecting tasks and withdrawing from all social contact. Other times avoidance is very subtle—for example, when a client is quite active and yet his or her life doesn't feel rewarding.

There are many examples of avoidance in Alicia's experience, and such avoidance patterns are connected closely to Alicia's struggles with overcoming depression. The session described at the beginning of this chapter alludes to both primary and secondary problems in the case of Alicia. Alicia's depression was triggered by the primary problems of being laid off from work, losing her condo, and not being able to find permanent employment after months of looking. It is easy to see how these problems are significant losses for Alicia and how they contributed to a less rewarding life. Because Alicia now works in a less desirable job and dwells in a less desirable home environment, her daily life is filled with more hassles and negativity, which also contribute to making life less rewarding. Although these life events were often unavoidable and beyond her control, Alicia coped with them through avoidance behaviors that contributed to greater depression. Commonly, however, people are not always able to respond functionally to primary problems and the feelings these problems evoke, and they engage in patterns of coping that are not effective in solving the primary problems and the related emotions. In the context of feeling depressed, this is typically a pattern of withdrawal and avoidance, and increasingly a narrowing of the activities in one's life (Lewinsohn, 1974). In effect, depressed persons become disengaged with many or all elements of life that once provided reward.

In Alicia's case, she began to avoid contact with almost all of her friends, stopped looking for a new job, and ceased doing things she used to enjoy like gardening or reading books. These avoidance patterns then became secondary problems, and she ended up stuck in a job she hates, with little social support, and engaged in few, if any, enjoyable activities. Alicia's pattern perfectly illustrates Principle 2 of BA, that "changes in life can lead to depression, and short-term coping strategies may keep people stuck over time." Staying in bed and avoiding social contact are common avoidance patterns; other examples of secondary problems include inhibiting emotional experience with alcohol or other addictive behaviors, constantly subordinating one's needs to those of another (such as a spouse), and staying in an unsatisfying relationship because of the fear of being alone.

These examples illustrate how avoidance patterns are often subtle and complex behavioral patterns that are not always immediately evident. For Beth, it was critical to identify the major avoidance patterns that perpetuated Alicia's depression and to begin to target these with active problem solving.

Validating the Natural Tendency to Avoid and the Challenge of Change

There are many good reasons why clients get stuck in the vicious cycle of depression and validating the difficulty of breaking entrenched patterns is necessary in helping move clients from avoidance to activation. When the avoidance is subtle, complex, or seemingly intractable, clients and therapists can become discouraged with incomplete homework assignments or the failure to carry out tasks that have been discussed at length in a session. The importance of the therapist's validating the client's difficult struggle as well as remaining hopeful and encouraging cannot be overstated. We often remind ourselves of Principle 8, which urges therapists to "Emphasize a problem-solving empirical approach, and recognize that all results are useful."

Another common response gleaned from Alicia's dialogue is the frequent question "Why am I so stuck? I should be able to do something to just get out of being stuck." In these situations validation can be an effective intervention and serve as a starting point for activation. Let's return once again to the dialogue between Alicia and her therapist, Beth, to illustrate some of the ways in which a therapist can validate the struggle of overcoming avoidance and in so doing help to promote change.

BETH: Alicia, I'm sure there are very good reasons for why you're stuck and not getting yourself out of your present state. Help me to understand what takes place for you when you're feeling down. You said that often on weekends and weekday evenings you lie in bed and "mindlessly" thumb through magazines. What would "unstuck Alicia" look like?

ALICIA: Probably getting up and calling a friend or going online to look for jobs. Something like that. Exactly what I'm not doing, I guess.

BETH: I think you're right; those are the very things that are extremely difficult right now.

ALICIA: Yes, plus my apartment's a complete mess, and I don't have any healthy food in the house. I'm really not taking care of myself very well.

BETH: Alicia, do you sometimes think about getting up and doing any of those things when you're lying in bed, or do you sometimes get up and attempt to do some of them? What do you notice then?

ALICIA: Well, sometimes when I think about getting up or even start to do so, it feels like a monumental effort, and I start to feel even more tired. The hopeless thoughts that "there's no use trying" return, or I start to feel anxious if I consider calling a friend other than Ellen. Even with Ellen I feel kind of guilty—she must get burned out on me for being such a disaster all the time. So then I just make either a half-hearted attempt or I make up an excuse to just go back to bed.

BETH: Well, I can understand, given how hard that sounds. Tell me, what happens to those feelings of fatigue and anxiety and the thoughts of hopelessness when you go back to or stay in bed?

ALICIA: Well, you know, I never really considered it before, but now that I think about it they kind of go away for a while. Sometimes I even feel a little relieved that I'm not really even going to make the effort that day.

BETH: Exactly, Alicia. That's a good example of the way in which you are feeling "stuck" and how it's so hard to move yourself forward. Remember when we talked about the rationale for therapy? We discussed the fact that when people get depressed they tend to withdraw and avoid things either because approaching them doesn't result in reward or because doing so ends up being punishing. I think that's what's happened with you and your job search and your living situation. I think it's really natural that you would be pulling away after all the struggles with your job and losing your home. The problem in this situation, however, is that you're more likely to continue avoiding these things in the short run because they're so hard and because when you do avoid them you get some relief. And, then, you're stuck—if you avoid them, you can feel a little better in the short run, but you're more down and stressed in the long run. I'm wondering if this is a pattern that has become pretty well established. What do you think?

In these ways, the therapist illustrates and validates for Alicia how it is that behavioral patterns can come under the influence of aversive control, which ultimately makes them more difficult to change. Beth simultaneously highlights for Alicia the tenacity with which avoidance patterns can persist and the importance of targeting them in order to take steps toward change.

It is often difficult for therapists to effectively validate the power of avoidance and the challenge of change. First, American culture promotes a do-it-yourself, pull-yourself-up-by-your-bootstraps mentality. Reaching out and accepting help is not encouraged and has likely been punished in the past. Although the client in your office has taken the step to seek help by initiating therapy, it's likely that the attitude of "Just do it!" is still very much ingrained.

Second, depressed clients experience very real difficulties in solving problems. Emerging neuropsychological literature suggests that there may be impairment in particular cognitive capabilities in depressed patients as compared to nondepressed patients. Fossati, Ergis, and Allilaire (2001) found that problem-solving abilities were impaired in people with major depression when they were compared to people who were not depressed. Impairment in decision making and the ability to carry out tasks has also been found in both patients with mania and those diagnosed with depression (Murphy et al., 2001), and problems with executive functioning skills and problem solving may be particularly evident among depressed patients who have suicidal ideation (Marzuk, Hartwell, Leon, & Portera, 2005). This literature supports the idea that clients need assistance with systematically tackling their problems and determining how to best proceed.

Addressing directly both the values of our culture and the vulnerabilities of being depressed is often helpful. Sharing the foregoing information with clients in an understandable way can be tremendously validating. A therapist can simply say: "A lot of people think that people should be able to overcome depression by just deciding to fix whatever problems are going on in their lives. There is emerging research, however, that suggests that the ability to solve life's problems is actually more difficult when a person is depressed. Depression has an effect on what we call executive functions, or, put more simply, depression impairs a person's problem-solving skills."

For this reason, we also return again and again to Principle 7, "Act as a coach." We emphasize strongly the need for a coach in undertaking something very difficult such as overcoming depression. Most people agree about the importance of a coach in learning a new or complicated skill, and we tell clients consistently that learning BA is no different. We explain that clients are the experts on their lives and their experience, and the BA therapist is an expert in solving problems, setting goals, breaking down tasks, defining problems concretely, and generating and evaluating solutions. The long-term goal is to teach clients these skills to the point of mastery so they can ultimately be their own coach. However, the learning process can advance at a slow pace and typically requires working closely in tandem, especially early in therapy.

In summary, validation is an important and useful tool in the process of helping clients counter avoidance and move toward activation. Validation helps clients feel like their therapist "gets" just how stuck they feel. It also helps clients understand for themselves why it may have been so hard to move forward on their own. For many clients, validation tends to reduce shame and anxiety, which in turn facilitates collaboration and the process of receiving help (Warwar, Links, Greenberg, & Bergmans, 2008). Table 6.1 provides a brief summary of reminders why validating clients' experience is so important when it comes to avoidance.

BA Problem Solving and Avoidance Modification

The first step in modifying avoidance is to define the problem behavior in specific concrete behavioral terms. For example, a problem stated as "I can't get anything done" is not described concretely enough to lead to a reasonable solution. It would not be satisfactory to simply say "Go out and finish some tasks." A more concrete definition might be: "Early on weekday mornings when I'm getting the kids ready, I look at the bills on my desk and I feel overwhelmed. Last Tuesday and Wednesday I got so upset that I just closed the door to my office and went down the hall and watched TV. I didn't return to the office

TABLE 6.1. Understanding the Power of Avoidance

It may be helpful for therapists to keep in mind the following simple facts about avoidance when working to validate a client who avoids, withdraws, or "escapes" a lot. These facts may help therapists find ways to understand their clients and may help to minimize therapist frustration or hopelessness.

- People tend to avoid when attempts to solve problems or otherwise engage their environment are not reinforced or are in some way punished.

- When a given behavior is negatively reinforced—through the avoidance of or removal of something aversive (escape)—the likelihood that people will continue to engage in this behavior increases.

- Increased effort to overcome fatigue, poor concentration, or other depressive symptoms is needed to activate and to be productive when depressed. For most people, the increased effort when depressed is aversive; to the extent that the avoidance of this is negatively reinforcing, it is more likely to recur.

- Cognitive impairment with regard to problem solving is an empirically supported phenomenon for people with depression. People who are depressed simply may not be able to engage successfully in the task of problem solving without help.

- It is difficult to counter avoidance and activate oneself when depressed. The contextual features of depression make it so. Depressed clients are acting in a way that feels natural and need coaching to counter avoidance and get activated because activating oneself may feel fake or unnatural in a depressed state.

From *Behavioral Activation for Depression: A Clinician's Guide* by Christopher R. Martell, Sona Dimidjian, and Ruth Herman-Dunn. Copyright 2010 by The Guilford Press. Permission to photocopy this table is granted to purchasers of this book for personal use only (see copyright page for details). Purchasers may download a larger version of this table from the book's page on The Guilford Press website.

to get other work completed because I couldn't stop thinking about those bills sitting there in the office. I sat around watching television until I noticed that it was time for the kids to come home from school! When I don't work, I don't have anything to submit for payment, and the cycle of having no money to pay those darn bills continues." The vague problem of not getting anything done has been transformed into something that includes the timing and frequency of the problem (two particular weekday mornings), the duration (the entire day, on both days), and the topography (leaving the office, watching television, avoiding work). Defining a problem in behavioral terms is the first step to solving it.

Often the activity chart is a good resource for defining prevalent problems in clients' lives. Once several problems have been identified, patterns may emerge. Alicia, for example, described that her lack of social connections was a major problem. This level of detail was not sufficient; so, Beth helped Alicia begin to identify the specific problems that needed to be solved in order to reconnect with some of her friends. In particular, it became clear that Alicia was hesitant to engage with her friends for fear that they would be put off by her depression. For instance, a former college friend, Terry, was in town and had called Alicia, asking if she wanted to have lunch. Alicia and Beth discussed the potential benefits of going to lunch, but Alicia was quick to add: "I just see us having this miserable lunch. She will ask how I am, and I know I'll tell her about how awful everything is, and I'll be a mess. I can't talk about this stuff without getting really upset, and I know it would freak her out. Terry will end up going home and telling everyone about how my life has fallen apart." Working together, Beth and Alicia clearly defined Alicia's problem as "I want to have dinner with my friend, but I don't want to talk too much about my depression." Avoiding friends out of a fear of burdening them appeared repeatedly in Alicia's activity charts and was a notable pattern among her problem behaviors.

Once a problem is defined, it is possible to work on solutions. A major role of the therapist in BA is to aid the client in generating and evaluating a range of solutions. Beth worked with Alicia, for example, to brainstorm a number of solutions that included "only talk about happy topics," "be honest, but don't dwell on the depression," "interview the friend, and don't let her ask any questions," and "plan for topics to focus on during the lunch." As mentioned above, the therapist also holds the responsibility for helping to evaluate the solutions. Alicia and Beth discussed the pros and cons of the possible solutions generated and decided that a combination of two had potential. Alicia stated the solution as "I will prepare some topics that I can discuss so that I don't dwell on my depression, and I will be honest during the lunch and not pretend like all is well."

Once a solution is identified, the therapist works with the client to structure a specific activation task for homework. Strategies that have been discussed in previous chapters such as managing contingencies, increasing engagement with natural reinforcers, grading tasks, and scheduling tasks may all be used as means for solving problems. Alicia and Beth realized they would have another therapy session before her friend would actually arrive; so, Alicia's homework was to contact the friend to set the date and then to generate the topics for discussion. The two scheduled times for each of these tasks on her activity chart for the coming week. With other clients, it also may be helpful to do an in-session rehearsal. For example, practicing assertive behaviors in session may prove instructive prior to scheduling a between-session assignment.

Alicia came to the next therapy session with a list of topics for her lunch date with Terry. She had identified people from college she might ask about or about whom they could reminisce and a list of questions she could ask, including: "What is it like to live in the Northwest?" "How is your family?" and "What do you remember most about college?" As Alicia and Beth discussed the strengths and limitations of each of these approaches and questions, Alicia realized that she felt worried that she might still feel sad talking with Terry and would come across as "a mess" even if she were not talking about her recent life changes. Again, Beth encouraged Alicia to identify this as a problem to be solved. She and Alicia then generated a list of ways that she could respond skillfully to sadness, if it were to arise. Alicia noted that she could be aware of whether she was slumping in her chair and frowning or sitting up straight and making consistent eye contact with Terry. In case she was asked directly how she was, Alicia practiced responding without using the word *depression,* which tended to elicit tearfulness, and by saying "It has been a rough emotional ride for the past year." Finally, Alicia decided in advance that she would excuse herself to use the restroom if she began to feel sad or overwhelmed.

With this plan in hand, Alicia went to lunch with her friend. She was happy to report back to Beth that the lunch date had been a success. She actually laughed out loud when discussing a former professor's classroom antics and a ridiculous prank that some of their dorm mates had played on a resident adviser. Alicia said that she started to feel sad for a few moments when she thought about how happy she was then and how difficult life felt now. However, she followed her plan and shifted her posture to sit up straight and shifted the topic of conversation to recent events in her friend's family. Once she felt confident that she was not slipping into a blue mood, she "went with the flow," and she and her friend talked for 2½ hours.

TABLE 6.2. The ACTION Acronym—Therapist Version

Through these ACTION steps, therapists can remind clients of the key components of BA: to evaluate the function of their behavior, to identify when they are engaging in avoidance behavior, to remember that they have a choice in how they respond to situations, to integrate new behaviors into routines, to observe and learn from the outcomes, and to persevere with the process of change.

Assess the function of a behavior. In other words, the client asks him- or herself how the behavior is serving him or her. What are the consequences? Does the behavior act as a depressant? Is it inconsistent with long-term goals? Does the behavior act as an antidepressant? Is it consistent with long-term goals?

Choose an action. The concept of choice is important for two reasons. First, BA is a collaborative treatment. Clients and therapists work together as partners. Clients maintain a choice over the actions that they implement. Second, many depressed clients do not have a sense of personal agency or control in their own lives. Explicitly pointing out that they have a choice highlights their ability to exert control and influence in their lives. Clients can choose to increase or decrease specific behaviors.

Try the behavior chosen. Putting the plan into action is the heart of BA.

Integrate new behaviors into a routine. This is an essential idea to get across. After months or even years of depression, one instance of activating may not have a strong impact. Trying a new behavior just once is not sufficient for evaluating outcome. The cumulative effect of working from the "outside-in" and increasing activity is important. Repeatedly activating as new behaviors are integrated into routines can lead to improvement in mood and life context.

Observe the results. The hope, of course, is that integrating antidepressant behavior into a routine will improve the client's depression. We cannot know if this will be the case until the client has scheduled activities, chosen to engage, and then, after integrating the activities over several trials, we and the client observed what happens. Observing the results, learning from what worked and what didn't, and using this information to improve future action plans are all key parts of BA.

Never give up. In other words, keep going through this process. Developing a new habit of activating and engaging requires repeated efforts. Over time, these antidepressant behaviors can become automatic, even amid overwhelmingly negative feelings.

Adapted from Martell, Addis, and Jacobson (2001, pp. 102–105) in *Behavioral Activation for Depression: A Clinician's Guide* by Christopher R. Martell, Sona Dimidjian, and Ruth Herman-Dunn (The Guilford Press, 2010). Permission to photocopy this table is granted to purchasers of this book for personal use only (see copyright page for details). Purchasers may download a larger version of this table from the book's page on The Guilford Press website.

Summary

As therapist and client work closely together, the therapist has many opportunities to validate the difficulty of approaching and solving problems while depressed. The BA therapist does this, in part, by highlighting avoidance—what it looks like and where it leads. The therapist explains often that avoidance is a natural and understandable part of depression but that avoidance rarely works in the long run because secondary problems tend to develop. In addition, the therapist also stands as a constant model for how to approach everything with a problem-solving attitude. Thus, whatever challenge or barrier presented by the client (e.g., not doing the homework), the therapist aims to respond with a focus on "What can we learn from this?" This stance of the therapist itself can be validating for the client, as he or she experiences a consistent nonjudgmental response characterized by perseverance and optimism.

In addition, therapists model a problem-solving stance in all of their responses to challenges and barriers that may arise over the course of treatment. One way to summarize this approach to problem solving is illustrated by the acronym "ACTION," as presented in Martell et al. (2001). Table 6.2 details the acronym from the therapist's perspective, and a client version is provided in Appendix 1h. BA therapists may teach clients to use "ACTION" to facilitate effective problem solving. Because primary problems are frequently unchangeable (e.g., the death of a spouse) or require a series of complicated processes to resolve (e.g., the multiple steps involved in seeking employment), the secondary problems maintaining the depressive cycle are most often the initial targets for change. In particular, the behaviors that function as escape and avoidance tools often are those tackled earliest in treatment. As we have discussed, the diversity of problems addressed by BA run the gamut from clients' neglecting to clean their homes to permanently being unable to secure employment.

One common specific problem to be solved is rumination. Depressed clients frequently spend a great deal of time ruminating about their problems, and such ruminative patterns can exacerbate depression. Ruminating keeps clients from full engagement in their lives and can thus serve as avoidance. Ruminating may prevent clients from actively seeking solutions to problems, or it may allow them to disengage from tasks that are uninteresting or overwhelming. Unfortunately, it also can disengage clients from activities that may provide reward. Ruminating is a process that is targeted for modification in BA. Table 6.3 provides therapists with hints for helping clients with problem solving and avoidance. In the next chapter we discuss how BA therapists help clients to change patterns of thinking that become problematic.

TABLE 6.3. Hints for Helping Clients with Problem Solving and Avoidance

When helping clients with problem solving it is often helpful to keep the following things in mind:

- Is teaching traditional problem solving appropriate in this case?

- Are you helping the client with a primary problem such as needing a new job?

- Are you helping the client with a secondary problem such as withdrawing from friends?

- Is avoidance a problem that needs to be addressed?

- Is the client acting to prevent something aversive, such as staying at home to avoid getting extra work at the office?

- Is the client trying to escape from an aversive experience, such as watching television to avoid stressful family interactions?

- Have you validated the client's natural tendency to avoid while helping him or her through the challenge of making changes?

- Is the ACTION acronym appropriate for this client in this situation?

From *Behavioral Activation for Depression: A Clinician's Guide* by Christopher R. Martell, Sona Dimidjian, and Ruth Herman-Dunn. Copyright 2010 by The Guilford Press. Permission to photocopy this table is granted to purchasers of this book for personal use only (see copyright page for details). Purchasers may download a larger version of this table from the book's page on The Guilford Press website.

7

How Thinking Can Be Problematic Behavior

Thinking is easy, acting is difficult, and to put one's thoughts into action is the most difficult thing in the world.
—JOHANN WOLFGANG VON GOETHE (1749–1832)

In her preceding session Alicia had committed to attending a small dinner party that Ellen had asked her to join. She successfully completed many components of the plan that she and Beth had developed. She carefully picked out her clothes the day before the dinner, thereby foreclosing on that particular excuse not to go. She also made a firm verbal commitment to Ellen, which she knew would make it less likely that she would back out. When the moment came, she attended the whole party. However, when she described the party during the following session, she related that she felt even more down than expected, experiencing a slight setback in her depression during the week.

When Beth asked about the details of the dinner party, Alicia started to cry. She acknowledged that she had made progress by attending; it certainly was different from the avoidance that had typified her behavior since becoming depressed. However, she felt like she was only going through the motions at the party. She didn't find the conversation enjoyable. The food was good, but she kept thinking that she should be enjoying the other people who were there. Throughout the evening she thought to herself: "I knew I couldn't do this. I'm too miserable to enjoy myself. Why am I always so depressed? I used to like these people, and laugh. Nothing ever works out. I shouldn't have come. I wish I could just not feel so down."

When Beth asked her what the conversation at the party was like, Alicia could not answer. She had been so immersed in her thoughts about being depressed that she had not really paid attention to the conversation.

Introduction

For decades behaviorists have been accused of ignoring activity from the neck up. Certainly behaviorism has assumed a strong antimentalist stance (e.g., Skinner, 1974); however, even Skinner (1957) tried to account for private verbal behavior. Although he did not succeed to the satisfaction of some scholars (Chomsky, 1959), his work leaves us with the important recognition of thinking as a covert private behavior that follows the same principles as overt public behavior (e.g., talking or telling a story). Accordingly, thinking is not a separate category of behavior that follows its own special rules but rather is "private behavior" and yet is subject to the same learning principles, such as reinforcement and punishment, as all public behavior.

BA uses this conceptualization of thinking as "private behavior" as a framework for helping clients who are caught in a web of negative thinking. As conceptualized in BA, rumination leads to two particular problems that are targeted to improve depression. First, rumination disengages one from one's environment and keeps the focus on internal thoughts rather than participation in the moment. Second, rumination prevents effective problem solving. The BA therapist works with the client to address these problems through a process of careful assessment, followed by the use of behavioral strategies including highlighting the consequences of rumination, problem solving, attention to sensory experience, refocusing on the task at hand, and distracting oneself from ruminative thoughts. The BA conceptualization of rumination in depression and the processes of both assessment and intervention are described in detail.

Rumination and Depression

Aaron T. Beck broke new ground when he focused during the 1960s on the importance of negative thinking among depressed clients.

Beck proposed that such negative thinking was not only a symptom but also perhaps a cause of depression. While the causal nature of negative thoughts has been disputed (Hayes & Brownstein, 1986), the idea that there are characteristic ways of thinking when people are depressed has been widely accepted. Clearly, it is important to address such negative thinking in the treatment of depression.

BA approaches negative thinking or rumination in a manner consistent with behavioral principles. Thinking can be understood as following principles similar to those for overt public behaviors. Certain thoughts and styles of thinking are reinforced, whereas others are punished. Words and ideas become paired with various emotional experiences and can evoke both positive and negative emotions. Words spoken publicly clearly have an impact. For example, when one calls someone an "idiot," there is an emotional consequence for both the speaker and the recipient. Likewise, if one silently calls oneself an "idiot," an emotional impact is likely experienced. Such public and private speech also can have an emotional impact long after the moment it occurs. It is in the nature of language that our words, and the stories we tell ourselves about our lives, allow us to reexperience emotions over and over again (Hayes, Barnes-Holmes, & Roche, 2001).

BA emphasizes the process by which clients engage in negative thinking by focusing on the antecedents and consequences of negative thinking and the context in which it occurs. For example, what happened before the client began thinking in this way? What happened after? Did it lead to effective problem solving (e.g., defining a problem, generating solutions, and arriving at a decision on how best to deal with the problem)? Or, does ruminating lead to a sense of "spinning one's wheels" (e.g., passively reviewing problems over and over without generating a solution)? Also, are there certain environments in which such unhelpful patterns of thinking are likely to occur? Alicia's experience at the dinner party was certainly an example of thinking that didn't lead to productive solutions. She kept thinking about how much more she used to enjoy herself before she became depressed. Rather than identifying a problem and figuring out what to do about it, her mind reviewed again and again how bad she felt, why she could no longer enjoy herself, and how she was doomed to lead a lonely and unsatisfying life. This is the essence of a process of thinking called rumination.

What exactly is rumination? The term "rumination" is a derivative of *ruminat*, Latin for "chewed over," and is used to describe thinking that consists of reviewing something over and over again in one's mind. It is to focus repetitively on one's experience of depression, including the causes and consequences of feeling depressed (Nolen-Hoeksema, 2000). Depressive rumination is typically focused on thinking about oneself and the condition in which one finds oneself, an ongoing perseveration on how badly one feels. It is to focus repetitively on one's negative internal emotional state without making plans, problem solving, or taking steps to make changes and relieve the distress (Nolen-Hoeksema, Morrow, & Fredrickson, 1993; Nolen-Hoeksema, Parker, & Larsen, 1994). Depressive ruminations are also mood-dependent—when one is feeling down, ruminations follow and are characteristically negative.

Susan Nolen-Hoeksema (Nolen-Hoeksema et al., 1993), a leading researcher at Yale University, has carefully examined the patterns of ruminative thoughts among depressed individuals. She and her colleagues have found that people who engaged in a passive ruminative style of thinking tend to be depressed for a longer duration and to experience more severe depression than those who used an active problem-solving style. Early research defined rumination as a unitary phenomenon; however, later work has clarified that there may be two types of ruminative processes, reflection and brooding (Treynor, Gonzales, & Nolen-Hoeksema, 2003). Both involve turning inward, but reflection entails cognitive problem solving whereas brooding entails passively rehashing the differences between one's current state and a contrasting optimal state. Although both are associated with increased depression concurrent with the rumination, only brooding is associated with feeling worse over time.

Similarly, Watkins et al. (2008) have highlighted the differences between adaptive and maladaptive forms of rumination. The adaptive type of rumination is characterized by concrete, process-focused, and specific thinking. The second, unhelpful type is characterized by abstract evaluative thinking and does not typically lead to solution-focused problem solving. Although adaptive rumination may be relatively common for everybody when a problem of some difficulty requires repetitive mental evaluation before coming to a reasonable solution, depressive rumination results only in an increase in dysphoria.

The process of ruminating keeps clients stuck in negative states and almost invariably results in disengagement from the environment. This assessment is consistent with the formulations of Lewinsohn (2001), who proposed that depression elicits a focus on the self that is repetitive but doesn't lead to problem solving. Clients can become caught in mental ruts, thinking, for example, "I feel down today— why does this keep happening to me? Will I ever beat this? This is just too hard." Such thoughts rarely have end points, they do not lead to effective problem solving, and the thoughts recur repeatedly. The consequence is a self-perpetuating process that keeps the individual stuck in his or her thoughts, less likely to find a positive, active solution, and more likely to be disengaged from other activities. Such sustained focus on internal feeling states may decrease any pleasure that can be derived from activities and may perpetuate depression by preventing goal attainment.

These patterns of thought were all too familiar to Kenneth, who sought therapy after being depressed for many months. Like Alicia's, Kenneth's depression began following the loss of an important job and subsequent months of unemployment. He had always considered himself a "survivor" and was surprised to find himself being diagnosed by a psychiatrist as having major depressive disorder. He took a job as a house painter making less money but was able to keep himself and his family afloat. Nevertheless, he had lost interest in most of the activities he once enjoyed, like biking with his kids, being the home repairman for little projects around the house, and he could no longer afford activities like attending baseball games. He felt fatigued all the time. When he arrived home from work, he spent very little time with his family other than to get a quick bite to eat. He then spent his evenings watching television. He'd gained 56 pounds over the past year and considered himself to be "a slob."

When Kenneth started therapy, he and his therapist developed activation assignments for him to increase experiences of pleasure and mastery. He left sessions armed with activation plans, but he found that each activity in which he engaged triggered thoughts about how fatigued he felt and how nothing seemed to help. In the mornings he thought about how down he felt. When he was at work, he thought about how he was forced to take such an easy job because he was depressed and no longer capable of working in a more challenging position. When he was home, he thought about how he used to enjoy spending time with his wife and two teenage daughters. Now it seemed that he didn't even care about his family. His eldest daughter was entering her last year of high school, and Kenneth thought about how much he was missing of her final year before heading off to college. He thought about the ways that the depression had stolen his life from him.

What should the BA therapist do with a client who is struggling as Kenneth was? In BA, two main approaches to rumination are used. Overall, the emphasis on working with ruminative thoughts is placed on the process, as we discussed previously, rather than on the content of such thoughts. BA therapists do not examine the validity of ruminative thoughts and do not ask clients to test the accuracy of their beliefs (as in other common approaches such as cognitive therapy; Beck et al., 1979). Rather, BA therapists target the process of ruminative thinking by looking at the context in which ruminative thoughts occur and the antecedents and consequences of ruminating. In particular, BA therapists focus on the ways in which situations may trigger rumination and what other opportunities may have been missed by ruminating. Furthermore, ruminative thinking can keep a client self-focused, disengaged from life, and caught in mental loops that do not lead logically to an end point. Helping clients become aware of these consequences may encourage participation in alternative behaviors. The BA therapist works with ruminative thinking by carefully assessing rumination and targeting it with a variety of behavioral strategies.

Assessing Rumination

Assessment is the first step in working with a client with ruminative thinking. In particular, BA therapists assess for ruminative behavior when clients report that they are engaging in activities but are not obtaining any enjoyment from them. In many cases, clients who are very active may appear to be doing exactly what they should in terms of overt behavioral activation but are not fully engaged in activities because their minds are elsewhere. It is important to assess differences between public behavior and private behavior because, although some clients appear to be actively engaged, they may remain disengaged from the activity because they are actually engaging in the private behavior of ruminating. For example, throwing a ball in the park with one's dog is a public behavior that looks like activation with potential high reward value. When a client says that he or she did not enjoy the activity, however, it is important to assess both the public and private behaviors to gain a fuller picture of the client's experience. Was she (say) tossing the ball while thinking that she felt miserable, that she would never feel better, and that this day in the park was so much worse than other days when she wasn't depressed? Tossing the ball *and* ruminating is a very different activity than tossing the ball and attending to her dog and the details of the park. This may explain the sense of "going through the motions" that many depressed clients describe. Indeed, the motor behaviors are present—going through motions—but the brain is engaged in a different activity, pulling attention away from the intended experience. To understand how to target rumination effectively, BA therapists must first review with clients the contingencies that maintain ruminating. Such assessment can then guide intervention. Here is an example:

BETH: Alicia, I'd like to know as much as possible about the situation yesterday when you were stuck in your thoughts about work. Can you tell me what was happening when you began to think that you weren't performing up to standard?

ALICIA: I was at my computer, answering e-mails.

BETH: Did you stop answering the e-mails when you started to ruminate?

ALICIA: I kept drifting off. It took me nearly an hour to do a task that could have taken 10 minutes.

BETH: Were you ruminating before you started to answer e-mails?

ALICIA: Yes. I actually started to work on my e-mails because I thought that might help.

BETH: That was a good try at getting active, but it seems like it didn't work yesterday. What were you doing before you answered the e-mails?

ALICIA: Watching television—some dumb daytime talk show.

BETH: Were you engaged in the show?

ALICIA: At first, I thought it would be good because they were going to have a segment on people who work from home, and I thought that would be relevant to me.

BETH: Did you want to watch that to distract you from ruminating?

ALICIA: No, I was okay before watching the show.

BETH: What happened during the show?

ALICIA: Before the segment about working from home, there was an interview with a teenager who is kind of a computer genius and has already graduated from college at age 17. That was what hit me. I started to think how lucky that kid was to be so smart and to have gotten that chance at 17 rather than having to go live with a whole new family. I was thinking that he was so dedicated, and I guess I was thinking that I was so lazy. It also just made me sad again.

BETH: Did you continue to watch the segment about working from home?

ALICIA: Yes, but I don't really remember it. At that point I was completely in my head feeling lousy.

BETH: So, the ruminating began when you were watching the talk show interview, right?

ALICIA: Yes.

BETH: Watching the show seemed like a good idea at the time but was actually quite painful. Do you think it is hard to know what might be helpful and what is not sometimes?

ALICIA: Well, I guess that watching talk shows is probably a bad idea. The very nature of them is a set-up for me to get upset about either the misery of others or my own misery.

BETH: You know that now and that possibly watching talk shows is a set-up. So, do you think it would have been easier to have worked on your e-mails had you not watched that show first?

ALICIA: It is possible.

BETH: Right, we don't really know for sure. I wonder if it might help to do some further work on scheduling activities like working on e-mails so that you aren't just doing it when you are feeling particularly down and ruminating a lot. What do you think?

ALICIA: That is probably a good idea.

Here Beth has followed the chain of events backward to ascertain when the ruminating began. The rumination was connected to a specific context, watching the talk show. It was a logical strategy to discuss an alternative to television viewing during the day in an attempt to prevent Alicia from being in the same vulnerable situation again. Also, given that Alicia ruminated in other contexts, the therapist would discuss other ways that she could respond to ruminating, including any of the strategies that we review in the sections that follow.

Often the consequences that maintain rumination can be as important as the antecedents that prompt rumination. Kenneth, who ruminated about depression stealing his life, said that he felt momentarily like he was doing something about his problems by thinking about how his life had been ruined. In this case, it became clear that his ruminating served as an attempt to discover solutions to his problems. Teaching Kenneth specifically to identify a problem and brainstorm solutions helped him to reduce the amount of time he spent ruminating.

For some clients, ruminating may function to decrease the experience of sadness. Maria's sister had died 2 years prior to her seeking therapy. She spent a great deal of time ruminating about the reasons that her sister had died so young, the negative effects of her death on her sister's children, and the emptiness of her own life without her sister. The psychologist Tom Borkovec (Borkovec, Alcaine, & Behar, 2004) suggests that clients with anxiety problems may worry in part because the linguistic process of worry (essentially talking to oneself) decreases emotional processing. Marsha Linehan (1983) elucidated the negative effects of "inhibited grieving" and this may also be present among some patients who ruminate frequently. These conceptualizations suggest that rumination may, at times, engage clients at a cognitive level and simultaneously avoid the emotional experience of sadness. Although these theories await future study with depressed clients, our clinical experience suggests that some clients, like Maria, tend to ruminate in part because it decreases the acute pain of grief. During therapy, Maria's BA therapist worked with her to identify activities that would allow her to approach the emotional experience of sadness, including reviewing photographs of her sister, talking about her dying process, visiting her nieces and nephews, and engaging in activities that she had formerly done with her sister. As she activated in these ways, her sadness increased temporarily, and her rumination and other depressive symptoms decreased.

In many cases, it may not be clear what function rumination serves. For some clients, rumination may continue because talking about sadness, loneliness, or other negative emotional states was reinforced at one time and has become a habitual practice even when it does not produce any relief from the current environment (Ferster, 1974). Rumination also may continue because there is an absence of other behaviors in which the individual engages. Some clients may be vulnerable to ruminative responses as a basic cognitive style.

In all of these cases, however, part of the task of the BA therapist is to help clients identify when ruminative behavior is serving them well and when it is not. As a heuristic to use in teaching clients to determine whether ruminating is helpful or not, Addis and Martell (2004) suggested using the "2-minute rule." They suggest that clients, when thinking about a topic, ask themselves after 2 minutes whether they have "made progress toward solving a problem" or "understood something about the problem" that they did not before. Also, they are to ask themselves if they are "less self-critical or depressed after thinking things over" (p. 97). Unless the answer to one of these questions is "yes," they suggest that "thinking" is in fact "ruminating," in which case they recommend an alternative technique to interrupt this pattern.

Targeting Depressive Rumination in BA— Don't Just Talk, Do!

BA Principle 9, "Don't just talk, do!," guides all aspects of therapist behavior. It is important to ensure that sessions maintain a focus on activation, limiting peripheral conversation and staying on track with assessing assignments, troubleshooting problems, setting new goals, and developing new activation plans. Of course, some amount of ordinary conversation is important to help clients feel connected with the therapist and to transition into more sensitive material. However, when therapists engage in too much passive conversation, therapy can become derailed. This is perhaps particularly true when working with highly ruminative clients. If therapists become immersed in simply talking about the content of a client's ruminations, without moving to action, they may actually risk perpetuating such ruminative behaviors. Many depressed clients want to talk to their therapists about their distress, but just talking about problems can be a way to engage publicly in the same passive ruminating that clients engage in privately. Such interactions are not likely to lead to solutions.

Within this context of activation, there are five strategies in BA used to target depressive rumination, namely, (1) highlighting the consequences of rumination, (2) problem solving, (3) attending closely to sensory experience, (4) refocusing on the task at hand, and (5) distracting oneself from the ruminative thoughts. Therapists can rely on their knowledge of a particular client and their functional analysis of the client's rumination when choosing one of these particular interventions. Each of these strategies will be explained in detail.

Highlighting the Consequences of Rumination

The BA conceptualization is a useful tool in highlighting the consequences of rumination. Therapists can demonstrate to clients that rumination is a secondary problem behavior that may make their depressive symptoms worse and may lead to increased problems in their environment. For example, when a client is ruminating about someone declining an invitation for coffee rather than offering a different time to the same individual or asking someone else out for coffee, the client's mood may worsen and social isolation may increase. This was the case with Charlie, and he and his therapist Tom discussed the consequences of his ruminations.

TOM: What happened when you asked Melissa to have coffee with you last Thursday?

CHARLIE: She turned me down. I figured she would. I couldn't believe it. I've been bummed about it all week.

TOM: Tell me about that, being bummed all week.

CHARLIE: Well, I can't get it out of my mind. It was just coffee. I wasn't asking her on a date, or to marry me—all I wanted to do was have a friendly exchange like you and I had discussed in therapy.

TOM: So, it has been playing over and over in your mind?

CHARLIE: Yes, all week.

TOM: What has been the result of playing this over in your mind or ruminating about this?

CHARLIE: I've definitely felt worse.

TOM: I was thinking the same thing, Charlie. Did the ruminating keep you from doing anything else that you had planned?

CHARLIE: Well, you and I had discussed having a "Plan B" in case Melissa wasn't available, and I never got to that point.

TOM: Because you were ruminating?

CHARLIE: At first I didn't ask her for a rain check because I felt hurt that she said she couldn't have coffee with me, but then when I kept thinking about it I stopped even saying "hi" to her when I'd pass her desk, and I never invited anyone else to do anything over the weekend. I just stayed at home, feeling miserable and thinking about how I'll never have friends, especially women friends.

TOM: This week sounds really tough. And at the same time, it seems like there is a lot we can learn from it. It seems pretty clear that brooding led to feeling a lot worse.

CHARLIE: Definitely.

TOM: It's interesting, when you were brooding, you were more likely to pull away from people around you and more likely to isolate, and you ended up feeling worse.

CHARLIE: Yes, that's right; I think that is pretty typical for how this goes, too.

In this situation, Tom highlighted the negative consequences of ruminating, helping Charlie identify the precise ways in which ruminating was connected to his mood and life context. At other times, therapists may elect to highlight the consequences of not ruminating, emphasizing the ways in which action as opposed to rumination can lead to better problem solving, more dependable goal achievement, and improved mood.

Highlighting consequences may serve a motivational function in encouraging clients to engage in alternative behaviors to ruminating; it also teaches clients a strategy to use when ruminating. As discussed above, it is important to engage clients in the process of assessing ruminating behavior. To help clients highlight the consequences of their own ruminative behavior, clients can be encouraged to ask themselves, "Is this way of thinking useful for me right now?" Most often, clients come to recognize that the consequences of ruminating are maladaptive. For some clients, this awareness of aversive consequences itself can shape behavior, and activation is increased. Other clients develop awareness of the negative consequences of ruminating but still feel stuck in the endless mental looping. For such clients, additional targeting of specific active responses will be important.

Problem Solving

We discussed the strategies of problem solving in Chapter 6. Problem solving is a natural counter to ruminative thinking. The role of the BA therapist often is to help the client define the problem that is a focus of ruminative thinking and to outline steps toward active problem solving. Together, the therapist and client identify the issue about which the client is ruminating and define a concrete problem to be solved. Then they generate and evaluate some possible solutions and develop specific steps to help the client experiment with change. As we have discussed, the BA therapist and clients work on solving a wide range of problems, ranging from challenging interpersonal problems to pragmatic employment problems. Solving contextual problems thus can provide a skillful response to rumination by eliminating the triggers for such rumination. At times, careful assessment of the problem may suggest that no solutions are readily available and that the best strategy may be to practice tolerating a difficult context. For example, if one is ruminating about the results of a medical test, which are supposed to be delivered any day but over which one has little control, the BA therapist may generate solutions for activities that are soothing or distracting in order to decrease a ruminative focus on troubling thoughts. In all of these ways, one of the primary tools of the BA therapist is problem solving; when a client presents with ruminative thoughts, as a first step it is often helpful to identify the problem and explore what solutions may be indicated.

Attending Closely to Sensory Experience

Many contemporary psychotherapy models have focused increasingly on the clinical application of mindfulness practices (e.g., Hayes et al., 1999; Linehan, 1993; Segal, Williams, & Teasdale, 2001). Mindfulness has been most commonly defined as "paying attention, in the present moment, intentionally, and without judgment" (Kabat-Zinn, 1994, p. 4). Whereas rumination pulls one out of the present moment, the aim of mindfulness is to stay engaged in the present. Mindfulness has been used with individuals with histories of depression to prevent future depression and, in this context, is frequently taught through a range of both formal and informal meditation practices (Segal et al., 2001).

In BA, we do not teach meditation. However, the practice of engaging in the direct experience of the present moment is central in targeting rumination. We refer to this practice as "attention to experience" exercises (Martell et al., 2001). Clients are asked to shift attention to the outside as well to what they are experiencing internally, in contrast to maintaining automatic focus only on what is happening inside their head. In other words, the client is invited to notice the sights, sounds, smells, and other sensations that are occurring in the moment. Attention to experience involves bringing one's awareness back to the elements in the context of the moment. The target of one's attention can include one's own sensory experience or what one is doing in the context.

For some highly ruminative clients being treated with BA, the integration of formal mindfulness strategies can potentially enhance treatment efficacy. For this reason, therapists are encouraged to familiarize themselves with mindfulness-based approaches to depression (Segal et al., 2001; Williams, Teasdale, Segal, & Kabat-Zinn, 2007). Therapists may provide clients with information about books on mindfulness, meditation practices, or yoga classes. Some clients may find these helpful in learning to reengage with the present rather than ruminating about the past or future.

Kenneth, whom we met previously, practiced attending to the sights, sounds, and smells around his house during dinnertime rather than ruminating while at the table with his family. His therapist, Miguel, helped him to practice noticing a variety of moment-to-moment experiences. Was the room silent? Did sounds from the outdoors come into the home, like traffic noises, bird songs, or the sound of wind or rain? What were the smells of the food on the table? What was the quality of the first taste of each bite of food that he took? As he developed the ability to direct his attention, with practice, at the dinner table, he began to add evening assignments of taking walks in his neighborhood in which he specifically took note of his neighbors' gardens, the colors of the flowers, and so forth. These assignments helped him to better engage with his family and to get physical exercise rather than watching TV alone. The key instruction to closely attend to the experiences provided him with an alternative to "going through the motions" of such activities while being trapped in his recursive mental loops.

Attention to experience and problem-solving assignments can be very effective, but, like all activation plans (as many people discover), they are hard to put into practice. When a client leaves with a between-session assignment to practice "attention to experience," it is essential to keep in mind the components of effective action plans. We have talked about starting small. This principle was central in Kenneth's therapist's mind when he introduced an attention-to-experience exercise.

MIGUEL: Kenneth, we've been talking a lot about how you feel caught in these mental loops in your mind. Does that seem right to you?

KENNETH: Yes, and it is a terrible place to be. I can't help it—I just feel so miserable.

MIGUEL: I understand that. Are you willing to try something different next week?

KENNETH: Sure, but you know I don't think it will do much good.

MIGUEL: I understand that as well. I'm wondering if you would be willing to give this the benefit of the doubt.

KENNETH: Yes.

MIGUEL: I would like to suggest that you practice a brief exercise that we call "attention to experience." The idea is to give your mind an alternative to that miserable mental loop your brain gets into. If we can train your brain to refocus on the here and now instead of its usual "looping," you stand a better chance of enjoying more what's in front of you and concentrating better on those things you need to, like work. Are you willing to give it a try?

KENNETH: I guess so. I'm not really sure what you mean, though.

MIGUEL: Good question. Let me give you an example. One thing to practice now might be focusing your attention on the various colors here in the room. Look around at colors and textures in the carpet or paintings. We can practice this together for a minute or two.

KENNETH: You want me to look at the colors for a minute?

MIGUEL: Yes, I realize it may sound a bit odd, and like all new activities, it may take a while to get the hang of it. Your mind probably will swing back to the usual patterns, and that's okay—it's all in the process of learning. When that happens, just come back again to noticing the colors, focusing on what's around you. If you notice any thoughts about how hard this all is, that's okay too—we're just starting here. When that happens, bring your attention back to noticing the colors in the room.

KENNETH: Okay, I'll try.

(*The exercise is conducted for 60 seconds.*)

MIGUEL: What did you notice?

KENNETH: Well, I noticed that there are little green flecks in the carpet that I'd never seen, and I really like that painting on your wall. I started to wonder who painted it, though, but I'm not sure that is what you were talking about doing.

MIGUEL: Yes, like I said, you can expect that you will quickly get distracted from attending to what's around you in many different ways. Your brain will pull you back into its habits of thinking, and probably also to that powerful habit of looping, very soon after you start the exercise. That's okay because your job is simply to notice that your brain has returned to its old familiar habit. Once you've noticed this, refocus your attention to what's in your immediate environment at home.

KENNETH: Oh, man, I'll probably have to refocus a lot!

MIGUEL: That's right, you will! Surprisingly, though, that's actually a good thing because what it means is you're doing a good job of noticing when you've drifted off, and you'll get lots of practice refocusing. With continued practice, you'll get more skilled at focusing your attention where you want it instead of where your brain just habitually drifts.

KENNETH: Hmmm. I guess that makes sense.

MIGUEL: How many times do you want to practice with this next week?

KENNETH: If I'm only doing it for a few minutes, I don't know—maybe three times?

MIGUEL: Okay. That sounds great. When during the week will you do this? Let's get that set so that you can initiate the activity according to your activity schedule.

Miguel has kept in mind the principle that change is easier if you start small. Rather than asking Kenneth to attend to experience for a whole afternoon, the assignment is for just a few minutes. It is also to take place at home, which should be an easier place to start, given that Kenneth is particularly unhappy at work and has a particularly hard time sustaining attention there. Miguel also treats Kenneth's doubts in a matter-of-fact way and explains to Kenneth how the strategy might be helpful to him. For some clients, asking them to attend to experience will be very different from the way they have approached life. It may indeed seem a little weird. Miguel also predicted that Kenneth might get distracted and begin ruminating, suggested a solution, and described how Kenneth would improve with practice. Miguel could also have asked Kenneth to write down what he noticed as a memory aid or to make him publicly accountable to the therapist for this activity, since Miguel could also ask him to bring in what he's written for them to discuss. Miguel also asked Kenneth to schedule this in his activity schedule, which increases the likelihood that he will follow through on the assignment.

Refocusing on the Task at Hand

This strategy is very similar to attention to experience since it requires clients to recognize when they are disengaged from a particular task. The difference between this and attention to experience is that the focus need not be on the moment-to-moment sensory experiences but rather on the particular steps of the task. Every time clients recognize that they are ruminating about something other than the task at hand, they quietly refocus their attention on some element of the task. This is often easier to do with a task that is more complicated or that has a series of steps.

Elizabeth, for example, worked as a mortgage broker. Although she was extremely isolated in her personal life, work had provided a place of solace for her. As her depression worsened, however, it began to impact her work. She complained to her therapist that she was much less productive and worried that she would lose the "one thing that really mattered" in her life, her job. First and foremost, she described her difficulty in focusing. She felt so bad that it was hard to get up in the morning and make it to work on time. Once there, she thought about how depressed she was because she didn't even enjoy her work. She also worried that she wouldn't be the top performer that she once was and that her standing in the company would be jeopardized.

She and her therapist decided that targeting these ruminative tendencies was key to overcoming her depression. Starting small, Elizabeth scheduled 10-minute blocks of time four times during each workday to practice bringing her thoughts back to the task at hand. As she reviewed financial records, she brought her attention from a focus on her internal state to the specific calculations she was completing. Although she found that she was distracted repeatedly by ruminative thoughts, she reported to her therapist that she did notice that she felt differently—"maybe slightly better"—during the times when she specifically focused on a task. Planning to do the 10 minutes four times daily also allowed her to practice with a variety of tasks. When she was on the phone, she listened closely to every word from the customer and worked to identify the essence of the problem that they were discussing. She occasionally asked the customer for clarification if she lost focus momentarily in the conversation, but overall she reported that at least she wasn't focused on how miserable she felt.

The activity itself is an important factor to consider in guiding a client to refocus on the task at hand when countering ruminative behavior. Clients may find it easier to practice engaging in activities that have a high reward value. For example, it is difficult to ruminate while maneuvering on roller blades or if one is skiing down a snowy mountain. Throwing a small cookie-making party for several friends' children may also be a naturally engaging activity. It is often easier to be fully engaged in the moment when tasks require focused attention, such as keeping track of the children, watching for spills in the kitchen, or playing physically challenging games with the kids.

Addis and Martell (2004) also suggest an acronym for clients to use as a tool for remembering to engage in the activity at hand rather than rumination. The acronym RCA—like the former electronics equipment manufacturer that General Electric took over during the mid-1980s—stands for "rumination cues action." Thus, when clients find themselves ruminating, they can remember "RCA" and make an attempt to engage in another activity that will increase the likelihood that they will not keep fixated on negative thoughts.

Distracting Oneself from Ruminative Thoughts

Refocusing one's attention on sensory experience and tasks at hand helps to disengage one's mental process from internal ruminative processes. Distraction also can serve a useful purpose in targeting rumination. The difference between the strategies discussed earlier and distraction is that, while attending closely to sensory experience enables me to focus on specific physical aspects of his or her situation, distracting oneself brings something new into the environment in order to disengage from the rumination process. For example, if one were ruminating while driving in a car, greater attention to experience would entail noticing such things as the feeling of the cushion of the seat against one's back, the hands on the steering wheel, the pressure of the right foot on the accelerator or brake pedal, the bumpiness of the road, the sounds of the engine running, or the colors of the surroundings. Using distraction, on the other hand, might add something new to focus on, something that is unrelated to the task at hand. In this case, one could turn on the radio in order to distract oneself from ruminative thoughts; or, one could sing a song that required effort to remember the lyrics. Both of these activities would be distraction because they don't require simply engaging in the current moment but rather adding something to the situation in order to shift one's mind from the rumination. Alicia tended to ruminate frequently at night, when she was trying to sleep. She found that attending to experience late at night, listening to occasional noises from traffic, and so forth made her feel uneasy in the darkness. She and Beth discussed distraction as an alternative. When she was in bed ruminating, she would shift her focus to the alphabet and think about all of the animals she could, beginning with the letter A. Alicia subsequently was pleased to report to Beth that she seldom got past the letter G before drifting off to sleep. They joked that thinking about a giraffe just prior to going to sleep was not a bad image to have! For some clients, distraction may provide an effective antidote to rumination. Table 7.1 lists a number of interventions that therapists may consider using when helping a client for whom rumination is a problem.

TABLE 7.1. Interventions for Ruminative Thinking

The interventions listed below can be used once the therapist has assessed that a client is spending a great deal of time ruminating or is not fully engaged in an activity but is brooding or ruminating.

- Highlighting the consequences of ruminating
  - Ask yourself: How does ruminating affect my mood? Is it useful to ruminate? Does it help me to solve a problem in any way? Does it have short-term or long-term benefits (e.g., reducing an aversive experience such as sadness) or costs?
- Problem solving
  - Define a concrete problem to be solved; generate and evaluate possible solutions; identify the steps to help experiment with change; put the steps into action; review the results and troubleshoot.
- Attending closely to sensory experience
  - Direct your attention repeatedly to the sensory experience of seeing, hearing, smelling, touching, or tasting in the moment.
- Refocusing on the task at hand
  - Identify what specific steps are needed to complete a task. Bring your attention back to one step at a time.
- Distracting oneself from the ruminative thoughts
  - Direct your attention repeatedly to a focus that distracts from ruminative thoughts. Do something active with your body (e.g., play with a pet, exercise) or with your mind (e.g., sing a song, go through the alphabet and list objects beginning with each letter).

From *Behavioral Activation for Depression: A Clinician's Guide* by Christopher R. Martell, Sona Dimidjian, and Ruth Herman-Dunn. Copyright 2010 by The Guilford Press. Permission to photocopy this table is granted to purchasers of this book for personal use only (see copyright page for details). Purchasers may download a larger version of this table from the book's page on The Guilford Press website.

Summary

Ruminating can become a troublesome and challenging experience for depressed clients. They can begin to feel that their minds are their own worst enemies. As depressive rumination often impairs full engagement in activities, rumination can undermine efforts toward activation. BA therapists target the process of ruminative thinking rather than the content. Rumination can also function as avoidance, keeping clients from facing difficult situations. BA therapists help clients learn several techniques for getting out of their heads and reengaging in the important activities in their lives. Highlighting the consequences of rumination can be used as a motivational strategy to encourage clients to stop ruminating. Problem solving, attention to sensory experience, refocusing on the task at hand, and distracting oneself from the ruminative thoughts all involve the client's actively practicing an alternative to depressive rumination.

8

Troubleshooting Problems with Activation

Great works are performed not by strength, but by
perseverance.
—SAMUEL JOHNSON (1709–1784)

Alicia felt discouraged about the dinner party. However, after working with Beth to target ruminating, Alicia was interested in putting some of the new strategies into practice and committed to attending a church service and staying after the service for coffee hour. Beth was eager to hear about the assignment and was surprised when Alicia did not attend her next scheduled session. She called Alicia after 20 minutes had passed and left a message reminding her of their appointment and expressing her interest in hearing about how Alicia was doing. She didn't hear from Alicia until 2 days later. At that time, Alicia called Beth, explaining that she had felt so down after going to work on Monday that she had retreated to her bed for the next few days. Beth replied: "I'm so sorry that things have been so tough, Alicia; it's great that you called today! I know how hard that can be when you are feeling down. Let's plan a time for you to come in so we can figure out what's been happening and how to get back on track. Does that sound okay?"

When Alicia arrived for her session the next day, she and Beth began to review the past week in an effort to pinpoint the factors that had contributed to Alicia's worsening depression. During this review, it appeared that Alicia's mood had been quite positive until Sunday afternoon, when she started feeling more down, and by Monday evening she was more depressed than she had been since the beginning of treatment.

Beth asked about what happened on Sunday before she started feeling more down. Alicia replied, "I'm not sure. It's hard to remember what I was doing that day."

"I think we had talked about your going to church that morning. Do you recall if you went?" asked Beth.

"Oh, yes, I did actually. Thanks. I did go and I even stayed through the service, but, after greeting the minister at the door, I just couldn't do the coffee hour. I think we had talked about my staying for that, too."

Beth was very interested in Alicia's experience of the assignment. She said, "I really want to hear about how you did in the service, since I know you were concerned that you might ruminate a lot then. I also am curious as to what happened at the moment when you decided not to go to coffee hour."

Alicia thought back to the service. She didn't think she had been ruminating a lot, but as she thought specifically about her experience she explained, "Well, I really didn't think I was ruminating a lot in the service, but actually that's not true. There were several times when I caught myself drifting, but the skills we talked about in our last session were really helpful. I noticed that I was feeling sad, and then I noticed that I was thinking about how much I wish I could feel spiritual again. But I had a lot of other things around me to focus on, like you suggested. I love that church just for the sanctuary itself. There is a beautiful rose window in the front of the church, so I would just focus on the colors of the stained glass. The sermon was also really good ... kind of just what I needed to hear that day. So, I would just turn my attention back to the rose window, or to the choir, or the sermon."

Beth was delighted to hear Alicia's report. "That is terrific, Alicia! You really put into practice what we had talked about, and it was helpful to you. That is great!" Beth wanted to hear about the rest of the activation assignment as well. She asked Alicia to tell her about the coffee hour. Alicia explained: "Well, I really was planning to go, right up until I greeted the minister. There were a few people there whom I knew, and they told me how good it was to see me."

Beth noticed Alicia's expression became tense at this point.

"What happened then?" she asked. Alicia went on: "I don't know. I felt overwhelmed all of a sudden. I just couldn't face talking about my job, or where I am living—you know, all the stuff I just hate in my life. It was like my feet were saying 'keep walking,' and I saw that it was sunny outside and headed out the door."

"That's really important information, Alicia. I'm curious what happened after that because you said that things really went downhill after Monday."

Alicia told Beth that Monday morning she had planned to stay home and telecommute but decided to go into the office instead. She was initially pleased with herself for making the decision and felt like she had accomplished a great deal to get out of the house at a reasonable time and go to work. The day had gone "downhill" because she discovered at the office that she had forgotten to complete work for a customer that had been promised the previous Friday. She had a telephone message from the customer, who was very angry, and the customer had also complained to her boss. Her boss had been polite to her but very direct, saying, "This work needs to be completed by the end of the day, and I hope you expect a long evening here." She did have to spend a late evening at work, but she also completed the work and delivered it to the customer.

The following morning, Alicia had felt exhausted and slept late. She had determined that she was not going to the office, so she slept a full 2 hours later than she normally would. Once she got up and took the dog out for a very short one-block walk, she was able to answer work e-mails. There was a "thank-you" e-mail from the angry customer, who also added that "the end result of this matter is fine, although your lateness has pushed back our ability to launch our new product by a full week." She sent an e-mail apologizing again for the lateness, copied her boss on the e-mail, and received a message from her boss a few minutes later telling her that she was "not to have any further exchange with the customer." At that point, Alicia returned to her bed, wanted to cry, and ruminated about her failures. She had stayed in bed through her therapy appointment, and when she listened to Beth's message she felt even worse. She waited 2 days before calling Beth because she felt ashamed about the failure at work as well as for missing her appointment.

When Alicia recounted these events in her session, Beth said: "I'm so glad you are here today, Alicia. What a hard week it has been!

It is terrific that you called and that you came in today. I know that is hard to do." Alicia was surprised that Beth wasn't frustrated with her. Beth smiled warmly, adding, "Perhaps we should put what happened at church and at work on our agenda to talk about further?" Alicia looked at her feet, acknowledging, "I had a feeling you were going to say that. I guess we should."

Introduction

Invariably, stumbling blocks arise during the course of activation, and this chapter examines the use of troubleshooting to navigate through these situations. As Principle 10 states, "Troubleshoot possible and actual barriers to activation." Troubleshooting is essential to address the types of problems that commonly occur when developing and implementing activation plans with depressed clients. "Troubleshooting" is used here specifically to mean two types of the "problem-solving" strategies discussed in Chapter 6. First, troubleshooting can occur once a solution or action plan has been proposed and additional assessment is undertaken to maximize the likelihood that the client will carry out the proposed plan. Second, troubleshooting may include efforts to debrief the client about what happened that may have interfered with an activation assignment that did not go as planned.

The heart of troubleshooting involves conducting a behavioral assessment and identifying possible solutions for the client to integrate in a subsequent assignment, and these tasks will be a central focus of this chapter. At the same time, the style and stance that the therapist adopts when troubleshooting also are critical. Thus, we first turn to the ways in which the therapist can approach problems that arise in order to facilitate effective troubleshooting.

The Challenges of Activation

Therapists may have the following ideal situation in mind when they assign homework to their clients. The client comes into the following session saying: "I did all my homework, and you know what? All of your interventions and assignments helped! I could do the assignments, I felt better by doing them, and I had more motivation to keep going. I'm ready to tackle more!"

These are not typically the sentiments of clients who are depressed, particularly in the early phases of therapy. Closer to reality is the frustration and discouragement that clients encounter when attempting to make behavioral changes in these circumstances. Clients typically feel guilt (or shame) when they have not completed their homework or have done something that runs counter to convention (e.g., missing work), especially when there are repeat offenses. Clients want to make changes, but often mood-dependent behavior gets the best of them. As a result, assignments often are not completed, and sessions may be missed if clients feel discouraged or ashamed of the challenges that they experience.

At such times, mood-dependent behavior can also get the best of therapists. It can be easy to feel discouraged or frustrated when depressed clients do not complete assignments, particularly when the therapist feels confident that such assignments would be helpful if completed. It can be very easy to blame clients for lack of progress, citing pathology such as "Axis II issues" or labeling clients as "help-rejecting" (otherwise known as clients who like to say "Yes, but ... "). While some clients do, in fact, meet the criteria for Axis II disorders, accurate diagnosis and the implications of multiple diagnoses for treatment planning are certainly important. At the same time, it is sometimes too easy for therapists to feel overwhelmed and frustrated and to fall into using nonbehaviorally descriptive judgments about clients—that one client is just manipulative or another wants to remain depressed. Unfortunately, such judgments not only fail to solve the problem but also contribute to burnout if the therapist's pessimism about the client is left unchecked.

The Therapist's Style and Stance in Troubleshooting Problems

Given the challenges of activation, relying on a variety of the core stylistic and structural strategies discussed in Chapter 3 can be extremely helpful. Structurally, obtaining the client's buy-in about the BA conceptualization can help ensure that activation assignments will make sense to the client. Maintaining the session structure, which keeps both the therapist and the client focused on activation, also will help to ensure that troubleshooting occurs properly. Ensuring that the client understands the therapist's reasoning and choice of various interventions can help provide a context for troubleshooting. The therapist's stance of validating the client—being nonjudgmental, warm and genuine when helping the client through problems with activation—can keep this process collaborative. Finally, while troubleshooting problems, it also is important to continue reinforcing examples of adaptive behavior, even if these behaviors are subtle or seemingly insignificant. In all of these ways, the therapist aims to adhere to Principle 8 ("Emphasize a problem-solving empirical approach and recognize that all results are useful"): approaching everything that happens over the course of treatment as an opportunity to learn and refine one's interventions.

A nonjudgmental attitude is essential when clients experience difficulty in completing homework assignments, make the same mistakes repeatedly, or engage in problematic behaviors. A nonjudgmental response that illustrates this principal might include saying something like "Hmmm. It seems we haven't solved this problem yet. Let's take a closer look at what interfered and see what we can learn." Or, "Okay, there's a good reason that this happened (or didn't happen) in this way. We must have missed something last week when we came up with this assignment, or perhaps a new problem arose. Let's take a close look and figure out which it is."

Each of these responses communicates that the therapist is not blaming the client for not completing the tasks and that the therapist is optimistic about identifying what got in the way. The emphasis remains squarely on "What can we learn here?" With responses like these from the therapist, the client usually relaxes a bit (he or she wasn't chastised for experiencing difficulty, after all!), and a productive behavioral assessment, as we discuss shortly, can be conducted to examine the point at which the difficulty with the homework or activity occurred.

As therapists review activity charts with clients, the use of a matter-of-fact tone is crucial. Requesting clients to record their activities and moods affords a privileged look into the client's life that, for some, may be uncomfortable. When planned activities did not occur or when a client has engaged in nonproductive or problematic activities, it's important for the therapist to comment on this without sounding disappointed or critical. This can be achieved by using a simple response such as "I notice you didn't get around to doing what you had planned on Saturday. How did that afternoon go for you?"

This acknowledges the event but also provides room for the client to talk openly about the day without needing to justify an answer to a question like "What went wrong?"

The emphasis also remains on identifying the contingencies that interfered with effective activation. The therapist may make remarks like "Oh, it's helpful to know [about a particular detail]" or validate what's been learned by saying "That simply is not a productive time of day for you, is it? Let's see if we can't find a better time and see if you have more success with the assignment this week." Through therapist modeling, the client learns that contingencies control behavior and that judgments such as "laziness" are unhelpful and tend to interfere with—not promote—effective problem solving. Once the important variables are discovered and validated, problem solving can be used to work around or modify activation plans so that progress toward goals can ensue.

The use of a matter-of-fact tone is also critical in carrying out analyses of problems that arise with activation assignments. For example, if a client says, "I don't know what happened. I did the exact opposite of everything we talked about my doing this week." A therapist using a matter-of-fact style might respond simply, "Tell me about it," communicating interest in a straightforward way.

It is also important for the BA therapist to adopt an optimistic style in responding to problems that arise in the course of activation. As we discussed in Chapter 6, BA therapists accept each problem as something for which one can help clients find a solution or a way to cope. Behavioral scientists know that change is difficult and frequently requires repeated attempts over time. Behavioral change may not be linear, sometimes occurring by taking two steps forward and one step back. A therapist who remains optimistic in the face of setbacks can be extraordinarily helpful to clients. Keeping in mind Principle 8's observation that "all results are useful" and point of view that behavioral change is a puzzle to be solved, both client and therapist can be confident they have what is needed to move the client forward toward their goals even in the face of frequent obstacles that may arise.

Such optimism can also give rise to a sense of persistence. The BA therapist adopts the perspective "If at first you don't succeed, try and try again." Often it is necessary to conduct behavioral analyses and generate solutions multiple times. Failure to persist when the client does not complete the task may result in the therapist's inadvertently reinforcing avoidance or getting caught up in the client's hopelessness. Also, failing to follow up on an assignment may result in a lost opportunity to reinforce any change that may have occurred. When working with depressed clients, it is critical for the BA therapist to look for opportunities to reinforce any signs of progress. Moreover, if a therapist stops asking about homework or directly addressing barriers that arise, he or she may begin to conclude that the client is "not able" to change in this way, especially if there are multiple attempts. Although this is a possible explanation, it does not provide useful behavioral information regarding what has actually occurred that may explain the failure. Without this information, it is nearly impossible to solve whatever problems remain. In essence, therapy gets off track here not because change is impossible but because problems are missed for lack of careful analysis of what may be interfering and because the therapist becomes frustrated or discouraged about the client's behavior.

Finally, clients in general, and perhaps depressed clients particularly, often assume they are at fault when a failure of some kind occurs. Adopting the attitude that there's a reasonable explanation for all behavior can lead to effective problem solving. BA therapists focus often on the impact of either learning or biology, emphasizing that vulnerabilities or deficits in either of these domains can interfere with success. This approach can help to reduce blame, shame, anger, and guilt behaviors, which otherwise could interfere further with effective problem solving. In essence, therapists deemphasize a stance of personal failing by reminding clients that there's more work to do in order to solve the puzzle of what needs to change the next time around in order for success to occur.

As BA therapists are working collaboratively with their clients, remaining open to the possibility that the therapist did not adequately grade the task or consider potential obstacles can also be useful. Therapists might reflect upon whether there weren't enough possibilities considered before a solution was attempted, or whether suggestions for the client were too elaborate. Reflecting upon this aloud with the client can also foster a sense of teamwork and help to counter the client's self-blame. Such reflection also extends to planning the assignment for the next week. The therapist and client can discuss what might come up during the week that would prevent the client from doing a planned activity. It is helpful to discuss both external barriers—such as planning to work in one's yard but encountering heavy rains all week—and internal barriers—such as waking up and "just not feeling up to it." When the client leaves with several alternative plans, the probability of success increases.

It is advised that therapists ask clients about problems or issues that may get in the way of completing a task as part of assigning between-session activities. Although these may be hard to identify prospectively, subsequent activity charts reveal problems that crop up and interfere with assignments. For example, if Alicia planned to buy mulch for her garden but had difficulty carrying the bags, she would need to figure out a way to get some assistance, perhaps by asking for help at the store and then asking another member of the pea patch to lend a hand removing the bags from the trunk of her car. She could plan to ask someone in advance so that she would be less likely to put off going to the store to get the mulch. Maximizing commitment to the activation plan is important. Often this can be as simple as saying "Okay, so we're agreed that you will call Ed on Monday and ask him if he'd like to work on the fence with you on Thursday after dinner?" At other times more discussion may be needed. The therapist and client can develop a list of reminders about the value of the activity that the client can then use later to help motivate him or her to undertake the activity. The therapist might ask the client to call him or her when the activity has been attempted or completed as an additional way of getting a firm commitment.

Finding Out What May (or Did) Go Awry

In their exceptional book on teaching people to change their own behavior through behavior modification (titled *Self-Directed Behavior*), now in its eighth edition, Watson and Tharp (2002) emphasize that successful behavior change requires good self-monitoring, a plan of action, and the ability to change some—or all—of the plan if it is not working. This type of flexibility is also necessary in BA.

Anticipating what might derail an activation plan at the time of assignment or identifying what did derail an attempted activation plan requires the use of ongoing behavioral assessment. As we discussed in Chapter 4, this requires testing hypotheses about what is maintaining depression and what behaviors may improve one's mood or life situation. If therapy isn't working, refining one's understanding of the problem, reevaluating the client's learning history with particular attention to skill building, or getting a better understanding of the consequences that may be reinforcing undesirable behavior or punishing desired behavior all become part of the problem-solving process.

Watson and Tharp (2002) also refer to troubleshooting as "tweaking" a plan. "Tweaking" suggests that only small changes may be required once a basic action plan has been outlined. And yet, even such small changes can be critical. Typically, behavioral assessments do not suggest that it is necessary to abandon the solution in its entirety after an initial try but rather that modification and persistence are important. This approach is consistent with teaching clients to make changes little by little over time and to integrate into a routine before deciding whether there is success or failure. Through behavioral assessment, clients and therapists can identify barriers that were encountered during implementation of the solution or aspects of the solution that did not work.

When barriers have been identified, the previous plan is "tweaked" to provide a strategy for overcoming the barriers. This process exemplifies how assessment continues throughout the therapeutic intervention. All activation assignments are treated as miniexperiments. The client can attempt the new plan, and upon reporting back during the following session the client discusses with the therapist the aspects that were successful as well as those that were unsuccessful in order to tweak the plan further.

Behavioral assessment always includes consideration of contextual factors that impact activities, such as the time, the place, and the other people involved as well as the consequences of the client's action that may either increase or decrease the behavior. Any number of barriers to completing a task may be identified, and there are several common problems that we have observed. First, clients may not fully understand an assignment to begin with. Second, clients may lack the needed skills to complete a task. Third, therapists may find that, while they initially thought certain tasks would be manageable for a client, in reality the task was not sufficiently well graded. Fourth, clients may not properly monitor activities or only partially monitor activities, providing insufficient information about mood and emotion to adequately troubleshoot barriers. Fifth, on occasion there are not sufficient cues in the environment to remind clients about assignments to which they have committed. Sixth, the contingencies may be set up to decrease rather than increase the likelihood of follow through. Finally, cues in the environment may be classically conditioned stimuli that elicit feelings or behaviors of which clients aren't readily aware. These common problems and their solutions will be addressed below. While the solutions proposed are not meant to be comprehensive, they can be used to guide therapists when helping clients to manage other kinds of barriers to activation.

Common Problems with Activation

Every client's experience of depression is unique; however, there are also common problems that arise as clients and therapists begin the process of activation. As clients undertake activation assignments, repeated behavioral assessments have revealed to us particular points when even the best of plans become derailed. Certain problems tend to crop up again and again, and it can be helpful to anticipate some of these problems ahead of time. The forewarned therapist can then troubleshoot these problems either when tasks are assigned initially or when problems are discovered in the process of attempting to complete the task. These obstacles and effective responses to them are our focus here.

Problems in Understanding the Assignment or Task

It might seem that it would be obvious to ensure that clients understand the task before leaving a session; however, in our experience this problem occurs frequently. When an assignment is not successfully completed, making sure that it was clarified fully in advance is a logical place to start. One way to prevent confusion from occurring is simply to ask a client to summarize the assignment after it is first assigned. Semantics is important here for two reasons: first, because the same words can mean very different things to different people; and second, because clients are sometimes too embarrassed to ask if they don't understand something. For this reason, the more concrete and specific the assignment is, the better. To say something like "Okay, so you're going to assert yourself with your boss at least one time this week" is neither as concrete nor as specific as saying: "Let's think of a way you can assert your needs with your boss this week. You said you wanted more specific instruction on the software task. Do you think you could ask him to set aside a certain amount of time for you this week to go over it in detail?" The latter is obviously much more specific in terms of being "more assertive" with the boss. More specificity could also include discussion of the best way to ask (e.g., via e-mail, voice mail, or in person) and determining when to ask. It is a good idea to ask the client to summarize what he or she has planned in order to ensure that the assignment is well understood.

Problems with Skills Deficits

While BA does not rely heavily on didactic skills instruction, it is important to assess whether specific skills deficits are either maintaining depression or interfering with enjoyment of a more rewarding life. This is another problem area that is easy to miss. Often clients are not aware of their deficits. Therapists can also miss such deficits because they assume that the required skill set is within the repertoire of most adults. Examples of potential skills deficits range from an inability to balance one's checkbook to an inability to assert oneself with the boss. There can also be skills deficits in emotion regulation, routine regulation, or in problem solving itself. When assigning homework of any kind, it can be useful to assess whether the client has the experience or know-how to implement the steps involved in the task. If the client indicates that he or she does but then does not complete the assignment, the therapist should have the client walk the therapist through what it is he or she actually did (or attempted to do) to see whether or not a skills deficit is present.

Sometimes a skills deficit is revealed only after multiple instances of failure to accomplish the assignment. The typical example of this is the client who repeatedly commits to something, has a plan to do it, has the apparent skills to carry out the plan, but then repeatedly fails to make sufficient progress on the plan. Basic self-management skills are a frequent and common target in BA. Breaking down tasks, sequencing them, estimating the time required to complete them, making lists, and tracking outcomes are mainstay preoccupations of BA with depressed clients. Persistently assigning the same task despite repeated shortcomings in its implementation may reveal a consistent failure to take into account that things often take longer than originally anticipated to accomplish. However, when repeated trials yield similar results, therapists may suspect that a skills deficit exists in estimating what can be realistically accomplished in any given time frame. Helping clients learn how to schedule sufficient time for unforeseen circumstances and to allow more time to complete each task (because things always take longer than one thinks) is a way to troubleshoot this common problem.

When working with depressed clients, interpersonal skills also are a primary target. Some clients, for example, may not know how to introduce themselves into a group conversation or when it is a good time to call people in the morning. Often depressed clients have difficulty in asking for what they want or making appropriate requests of people in their lives. Therapy sessions with such clients might focus on practicing being interpersonally effective and, in particular, assertive with specific people in their environment. For some clients, social anxiety also will get in the way and needs to be dealt with so the client can practice skills.

Finally, some clients may lack skills in regulating emotion and may find that hyperarousal interferes with the efficiency with which they process incoming stimuli. An example of this is when a client is so angry during an argument with a relative that he cannot follow the logic of the conversation and discuss a resolution. In this case, emotion regulation skills such as breathing, relaxation, or taking a timeout from an overstimulating environment to decrease hyperarousal can be taught. Conversely, some clients have distracted themselves from their emotions for so long that they have trouble identifying which emotion they are experiencing in any given moment, and crucial information that can inform an appropriate response is often missed. Teaching a client about the nature of different emotions and how to identify them often can be useful. All of these problems can be conceptualized as skills deficits to be addressed with skills training in the context of BA.

Problems with Grading Tasks

Ensuring that clients have the requisite skills to accomplish tasks may require teaching new behaviors and having clients start with the simpler aspects of complex activities. Additionally, assignments need to be realistic within the context of the client's life experiences. Principle 5 states that "change will be easier when starting small," and assignments may go awry because they weren't broken down adequately. Two ways that therapists can help to make sure an assignment is manageable are to grade tasks accurately (as described in Chapter 5) as well as to keep in mind that behavior change is usually difficult and progress can be slow. For various reasons, clients often overestimate what they can accomplish, and to the extent that therapists emphasize the importance of starting small, their clients are more likely to be successful in their endeavors. Success tends to reinforce the efforts of both the client and therapist and thereby to encourage additional steps toward positive change.

At the outset, clients do not always realize that a task is too difficult or overwhelming, and this issue is often the bugaboo of incomplete tasks. For this reason, hypotheses about incomplete assignments can only be "proved" by experimenting with grading the task, reassigning it, and assessing whether or not the client has more success. BA therapists remain mindful that some depressed clients hold expectations that they should be doing much more in their initial activation efforts. Some clients also romanticize their lives before becoming depressed, and they recall having done much more than they actually did. They can also make unfair comparisons of themselves with others whom they believe are accomplishing much more. Such comparisons occasionally include the assumption that those who apparently are accomplishing huge tasks are doing so with ease and without negative consequences such as increased stress, worry, or interference in other areas of life. The BA therapist does not question the validity of these assumptions but simply focuses on grading the task appropriately, saying to the client: "When we say that change happens in small increments, we really do mean small. I'd like to maximize your success in doing this task, so let's start really small. It's okay if you do more; I just want to be sure that you know that you will have succeeded in the assignment if you do this first step." Clues indicating problems with task grading include the client's feeling overwhelmed, discouraged, making multiple mistakes, or repeated failed attempts. When in doubt, it never hurts to break an assignment down into smaller steps, especially if it increases the likelihood that the client will return to the next session after having experienced some measure of success.

The Absence or Inadequacy of Activity Monitoring

Initially several problems may arise in response to an activity chart assignment. Sometimes clients simply do not complete any part of the chart. This failing provides therapists with an opportunity to conduct a behavioral analysis to understand and problem-solve specifically what interfered with the assignment. Noncompletion is a problem to address directly and immediately. It is critical to conduct an assessment of the factors that contribute to clients' not completing their activity charts.

Sometimes clients will say, "I don't want to put a microscope on how I feel because doing so just makes me feel worse so—why on earth would I do that?" Although this perspective may seem accurate to them, it also may be an example of avoiding something aversive in the short run that, if accomplished, would serve their long-term interests. Using a collaborative troubleshooting approach to this dilemma can help clients engage in the process of monitoring in a way that is not overwhelming. This can be done by either grading the task or changing the assignment such that in the short run the emphasis is placed more on recording activities and less on negative affect. It is also possible to develop with the client briefer or fewer monitoring periods, effectively grading the task of monitoring. Clients can be subsequently enlisted into a more thorough assessment of activity and mood once they become more familiar with the process of self-monitoring and feel less threatened.

It is important for therapists to remember that they aren't required to use a specific form or a prescribed format for an activity chart or self-monitoring technique for their clients. The goal is to create a tool for understanding the relationships between context, activity, and mood such that mood-related problems can be explored and improved upon while clients are ultimately brought into contact with more positive reinforcers in their lives. For some clients, doing paperwork of any kind feels like having school assignments or is intimidating. When clients don't like to complete forms, the therapist and client can discuss other ways to record the data when they are monitoring their behavior or when they are planning activities. Some clients might prefer to talk into a small audio recorder or even to use golf counters if they are collecting data on the frequency of particular behaviors. While there isn't an easy solution that works for all, therapists are encouraged to collaborate creatively with their clients to find a monitoring method that will be both effective and palatable to them.

Limited Information about Mood or Emotion

Another common situation is that clients bring the activity chart back only partially completed. Often clients will have recorded activities with very little variance in mood noted or perhaps no information about mood at all. In such cases, the client often reports, "I'm depressed all the time. Nothing makes me feel good." The therapist may emphasize that during depression subtle changes in mood tend to go unnoticed; this is a very common problem in the treatment of depression. Self-monitoring is an excellent antidote to this, as the monitoring process itself can increase clients' awareness of their own experience. Monitoring behavior can also have an impact on the behavior itself, since behavior often is reactive to observation (Mace & Kratochwill, 1985). The therapist can say something like "When you are feeling down, it is very common to not notice small changes in mood because everything seems so gray. From experience, I know that putting a microscope to your mood throughout the day will help you fine-tune your observations of subtle changes. Once this occurs, we can capitalize on these subtle changes by increasing those behaviors that tend to improve your mood and decreasing those behaviors that tend to detract from it." In such situations, it is often useful to practice with monitoring tasks in session, asking the client to walk back through the hours just prior to coming to therapy and identifying activities and associated variations in mood.

Problems with Cue Control

How often do therapists ask about homework, only to find out that clients have forgotten to do the assignment? This problem can be attributed to clients' not getting cued during the week to engage in the behavior they planned to do. In other words, the assignment failed to happen not because the client was apathetic but simply because there was nothing in the environment that reminded him or her to do it. Failing to complete the activity chart (or other self-monitoring tasks) and failing to arrive on time (or at all) for appointments are common examples of this problem.

Rather than ascribing negative motives to the client, the therapist should simply ask what interfered with the assignment. Clients don't always know initially why something did or did not happen and will either say "I don't know, I just didn't do it" or will feel compelled to try to come up with an explanation or motive because they think that's what they are "supposed" to do.

It's always safe to do a behavioral analysis of the chain of events for when the task *might* have occurred. A simple way to begin is to ask whether the client thought about or remembered the homework assignment at any time during the latest week, especially if it's a first-time assignment and/or the client is new to therapy. When asked specifically about recall during the week, clients will often realize that it simply never occurred to them to do the assignment once they left the therapist's office.

Depending on what the client thinks is more helpful, either a visual cue (e.g., put something by the door, bed, desk, or leave a Post-it in a prominent place) or an auditory cue (e.g., leave oneself a voice mail, set an alarm or timer) can be arranged so that the client is reminded of the task. It may be necessary for either the client or therapist to write down the assignment during the session so there is no confusion and to help minimize forgetfulness. One client, who tended to forget assignments because of his busy schedule and mild concentration difficulties resulting from his depression, would call himself on his cell phone during the therapy session and remind himself of particular therapy assignments. Clients who are more severely depressed may find it helpful to schedule a brief phone check-in with the therapist between sessions to help ensure that the plans discussed during sessions remain accessible to the client. Having a commitment to communicate with the therapist may increase the likelihood of completion as well, so the phoned check-in may well serve the twin purposes of enhancing memory and making it more likely that the activity will be completed.

Problems with Contingency Management

Not having an accurate understanding of the antecedents and consequences of behavior is another common problem that can get in the way of well-intended action plans. Poor behavioral specificity, poor assessment, or both can be at issue. Contingency management is nothing more than arranging one's immediate environment in ways that maximize the likelihood of desired consequences.

Suppose, for example, that the therapist reviews the activity chart and sees that her client gets a boost in her mood when window-shopping. A reasonable hypothesis to test is that window-shopping is a behavior to increase, given that it likely improves her mood and future excursions may continue to do so. This possibility is discussed with the client, and it's agreed that the client will go window-shopping three times over the course of the next week. The client returns with her activity chart, only to show that, although she did complete the assignment, her mood actually worsened each time she went window-shopping. This time, the therapist more carefully assessed the context of the activity, including the time of day and what occurred in the environment upon her return home. The therapist learned that this week (unlike before) the client went window-shopping in the evening before making dinner—which was her typical family routine—and the meal was delayed. When she returned home, she was met with cranky children and found herself feeling tired and overwhelmed. Learning about the context and consequences of the behavior provided information that the therapist and client could use to determine a more appropriate time of day that wouldn't deplete her or aggravate anybody in her household. This is a good example of where scheduling assignments can be helpful and troubleshooting problems ahead of time will also help to ensure that the consequences of a given activity or behavior will in fact be rewarding to a client. Troubleshooting the assignment in this case might simply be to ask: "Will anything get in the way of your going window-shopping? Is there anything that would make this activity harder or easier if you go at the time we have planned?" Troubleshooting provides an opportunity to generate some new activities to try during the week and revise others that are inconsistent with well-being or goals.

Occasionally problems arise owing to contingencies involving secondary gains of which the therapist is unaware. Unresolved legal suits or disability claims can potentially fall into this category. Discussing the difficulties of competing goals (e.g., feeling better emotionally and psychologically vs. getting a settlement) may help reduce the impact of the conflict. Clients in these dilemmas are not necessarily intentionally trying to mislead therapists in this regard; clients themselves can sometimes fail to appreciate all the contingencies that may impinge on a given behavior. Interpersonal relationships in which a client gets additional attention from his or her partner for behavior that is otherwise problematic (such as staying in bed) is an example of how contingencies can work against change for the client while remaining outside his or her conscious awareness. BA therapists occasionally invite the client's partner to a few therapy sessions to discuss these very issues and to enlist that important person's help in changing the contingencies.

Problems with Classically Conditioned Behaviors

Many clients who present with depression have suffered significant losses in their life, sometimes of a traumatic nature. A common response to trauma is that current situations can be cues for distress about the original traumatic event and are typically responded to with avoidance. Any variety of responses can be paired with any vari-

---

TABLE 8.1. Troubleshooting

When troubleshooting problems that arise in BA, therapists should consider the following guidelines:

- Maintain a nonjudgmental stance when clients have problems with activation.
- Consider contextual factors that have impacted activities and barriers to success.
- Assess possible problems with activation:
  - A client hasn't understood the assignment or task.
  - A client may require that the tasks be graded in a more manageable way to take the first steps toward change.
  - A client may require skills training prior to attempting a new task (e.g., assertiveness, time management, etc.).
  - A client may require specific training to complete monitoring tasks (e.g., recording adequate detail, identifying specific emotions or intensity of mood)
  - A client may not have sufficient cues to remind him or her of the assignment.
  - A client may have competing contingencies that get in the way of doing the assignment.
  - A client may have conditioned responses that interfere with doing the assignment (e.g., a client who had a difficult break-up with someone from a particular neighborhood may suddenly feel emotionally overwhelmed when attempting to follow through on an assignment to sign up for a class offered in a building in that same neighborhood because the neighborhood itself has become a conditioned stimulus for sadness, triggering memories of the loss).
- Does the plan require tweaking?

---

ety of cues that result in limited or avoidant behavioral repertoires. The urge to drink, for example, is often classically conditioned to such cues as specific people, places, or situations. Careful analysis of the antecedents and consequences of behavior will reveal whether a behavior is one that is an automatic response to a particular cue. For example, one client began an extended period of alcohol abuse each time she went out to dinner with particular coworkers at a local bar and grill. Giving in to the urge to drink may then be maintained by positive reinforcement via the intoxication that ensues or the increase in warmth and approval received from a drinking buddy. Negative reinforcement can also come into play here to the extent that drinking provides relief or enables avoidance of something aversive in the internal (e.g., mood states) or external (e.g., a negative interpersonal interaction) environment. Being aware that a problematic behavior is occurring automatically in response to some sort of stimulus or cue in the environment enables the therapist to use problem solving to see whether such cues can be modified through a process like desensitization or need to be avoided altogether in order to encourage more functional behavior.

Summary

Problems in activation are to be expected in therapy and are viewed as opportunities to learn more about the client. Table 8.1 provides therapists with suggestions for troubleshooting problems that may arise during the course of therapy. In our experience, the problems described in this chapter are fairly common and once assessed can be addressed effectively with troubleshooting. Without careful assessment, however, these problems can be easy to miss, and, as a result, activation plans can easily go awry. Anticipating and knowing how to assess for and approach these common problems can go a long way toward achieving successful solutions with clients.

9

Tying It All Together: Relapse Prevention and Beyond

The past cannot be changed. The future is yet in your power.
—MARY PICKFORD (1892–1979)

When Alicia had completed 18 sessions of therapy, she and Beth began to talk about ending treatment. Since the start of treatment, Beth had emphasized the importance of Alicia's learning strategies and making changes in her life that would help her feel better now and protect herself from depression returning again in the future. As they approached the 18th session, the focus on how Alicia could best care for herself over the long term became even more salient.

Beth and Alicia reviewed Alicia's reports of the severity of her depression since the start of therapy. Although her level of severity had fluctuated over the course of treatment, her scores on the Beck Depression Inventory–II were consistently in the nondepressed range over the last three sessions. Her scores on anxiety scales were still mildly elevated, but Alicia expressed some confidence in facing fears. She also described making frequent use of the skills she had learned as alternatives to ruminating. Overall, Alicia reported that she felt relief from her depression, was better able to manage her "down days," and was making important changes in her life. In addition to increasing contact with friends, she and a friend were considering moving in together in a nicer neighborhood. As a way to stay connected to

169

others, she spent more time at her office rather than telecommuting from home. Alicia was keeping up with basic housework, and she was taking her dog for daily walks. She also had developed strategies for dealing directly with her boss rather than avoiding feared conflicts. As work had been a major problem and Alicia still wanted to find a better long-term work situation in recent sessions, she and Beth began updating her résumé and brainstorming about ways to actively seek out new employment.

With respect to her future, Alicia reported a sense of cautious optimism about the future. However, she also knew that individuals who have had one major depressive episode were likely to have another, and she was concerned that she would experience depression again. As she and Beth prepared for the final phase of therapy, the topic of relapse and prevention became the primary focus. Together, they reviewed carefully what had been helpful for Alicia in therapy, including the new skills she had learned and the life changes she had made, and they looked to the future to identify possible areas of vulnerability and ways in which Alicia could cope effectively.

Introduction

BA follows a logical course over time. In the early sessions, therapists focus on presenting the treatment model and developing and refining the case conceptualization. There also is heavy emphasis on client self-monitoring, primarily with activity and mood-monitoring charts. The therapist and the client actively hypothesize what behaviors might be antidepressant and focus on bringing the client into contact with positive reinforcers in the natural environment. In this way, therapists and clients target directly the secondary problems, such as withdrawal and avoidance, that frequently maintain and exacerbate depression. Addressing secondary problems as initial targets can enable clients to break the cycle of depression so that primary problems are more easily managed. For some clients, these secondary problems may be the only targets of treatment; however, for many, primary problems, such as needing a new job, also are addressed in treatment.

Throughout the process of treatment, therapists act as coaches accompanying clients through the process of approaching and solving problems and making life changes. Together, therapists and clients structure and schedule activities that have potential for antidepressant consequences. Barriers to change invariably arise, such as the tendency for people to engage in avoidance behavior or to think in a ruminative fashion. Therapists approach such challenges as opportunities for new learning, adopting a nonjudgmental problem-solving stance. Thus, BA involves repeated application of the following elements: monitoring, structuring and scheduling activities, problem solving, and troubleshooting.

In our clinical research studies, these phases of treatment generally occur across a maximum of 24 sessions. Other related BA models have utilized shorter courses of treatment, such as 8–15 sessions (Hopko, Lejuez, Ruggiero, & Eifert, 2003). Over the course of treatment, it is important to maximize the likelihood that clients will maintain new patterns of activation and engagement following treatment. Thus, as therapy is nearing the end, it is often beneficial to review and consolidate what has been helpful and to anticipate future challenges that may increase risk for relapse. To this we now turn.

The Importance of Relapse Prevention

Given the recurrent nature of major depressive disorder, it is important for all treatments for depression to both reduce current distress and to provide protection from relapse. For this reason, relapse prevention is programmed into BA from the start and is increasingly a central focus of sessions as the course of treatment comes to a close. In this section, we review key components of BA that are relevant to relapse prevention. First, we discuss the emphasis on generalization, which is woven inextricably into the fabric of each and every BA session. Second, we discuss specific strategies the therapist can employ to address relapse prevention directly. Many of these strategies are consistent with the principles of relapse prevention articulated by Marlatt and Gordon (1985) for substance abuse and later adapted for depression (Wilson, 1992). Key strategies include identifying the ingredients of antidepressant behaviors, expanding activation to other life contexts, identifying and preparing for high-risk situations, and using booster and maintenance sessions.

Generalization

The transfer of training—or "generalization"—is an important factor in any behavioral treatment or program. When a skill trained in one context is generalized, that means it transfers to other contexts. Instilling the ability to transfer what's been learned in one context to another is a critical component in any relapse prevention plan. It enables clients to respond effectively when presented with new situations that may have once triggered depression.

Behaviorists often differentiate between two types of generalization, stimulus and response generalization (Sulzer-Azaroff & Mayer, 1991). Stimulus generalization occurs when the same response occurs in the presence of different contextual factors. For example, if William, who has a mild level of social anxiety and timidity, develops the skill to speak assertively with his therapist and then behaves similarly with his coworker and mingles freely at a party with several new people, we would say his assertive behavior has generalized to different stimuli. Response generalization, the second type of generalization, refers to instances when responses themselves change in nature over time and in varying contexts. For example, while William's behavior has generalized, he may have stated to his therapist very clearly, "I would much rather meet at 3:00 P.M. than 9:00 A.M. because it is better for my schedule." Later he may have said to his coworker "I've been meaning to ask you, if you could cover my shift for me on Thursday?" With the therapist, William was direct and to the point and this assertive behavior generalized to a coworker. With the coworker, he was less direct although still assertive. He then used the same assertiveness skills to introduce himself to guests at a party. Thus, the behavior generalized to different stimuli—the therapist, coworker, and party guests—but the topography of the behavior also generalized and looked slightly different in the different contexts.

Several methods exist for incorporating generalization into a behavioral training program (Stokes & Baer, 1977). A critical element to many includes using a range of modalities of training in different physical settings and with different people. Such methods support eventual generalization of the new behavior to more naturalistic settings (e.g., Martell, 1988). Because therapy takes place in a clinical setting (usually in the therapist's office), not in a naturalistic environment, training of this type can be challenging. For this reason, behavioral and cognitive-behavioral treatments such as BA place a great deal of weight on client homework assignments. The emphasis in BA is placed on what the client does in his or her daily life rather than what happens in the clinician's office. Through the use of homework assignments, BA incorporates training in multiple settings by asking clients to engage in specified activities repeatedly in a variety of contexts. Generalization is most likely to occur when activities are practiced in different contexts (i.e., at different times of day, in a variety of physical settings, with different people). In addition, integrating new behaviors into routines can facilitate generalization. Our experience with BA suggests that, as clients' ability to generalize adaptive behavior increases, the likelihood of relapse decreases.

Families and significant others can also be enlisted to help in generalization. Generalization is most likely to occur when clients' new antidepressant behaviors (e.g., going out with friends or accomplishing tasks at home) are reinforced by significant others and depressed behaviors (e.g., staying in bed) are extinguished.

Ingredients of the Behavioral Antidepressant

Encouraging clients to create their own personal handbook based on what they have learned in BA can help prevent relapse. We often think of this as listing the ingredients of each client's own personal behavioral antidepressant. For many clients, this handbook consists of a single sheet of paper that lists the various activities that they have found helpful throughout the course of treatment. Some clients may include a folder of their activity charts and logs. Clients who keep notes during therapy sessions can be encouraged to summarize these in their handbook as well. Appendices 2 and 3 provide examples of some questions that can help clients to summarize what they have learned over the course of treatment and that may help them to cope with the risk of depression in the future. As Figure 9.1 illustrates, Alicia's list included the key methods of activation that she had practiced over the course of treatment. Such handbooks should be tailor-made to fit the particular client, and the sample in Appendix 3 can be amended to fit the client's needs or preferences. The main task for the BA therapist is to help review the components of treatment that were helpful to the client, including particular principles discussed in Chapter 2 as well as specific strategies such as using "ABC" analyses

- What contexts increase my vulnerability to depression?
  Living in an environment that I don't like.
  Getting out of touch with friends.
  Working in a job for which I am overqualified.
  Being reminded of rough times that happened in the past and that I cannot change.

- What behaviors contribute to keeping the depression cycle going?
  Not calling friends or returning phone calls.
  Reducing my physical activity and telling myself, "I'm too tired."
  Slowing down on daily chores, especially cleaning my apartment.
  Telling myself, "This is totally overwhelming" many times a day.
  Avoiding social activities like going to church.
  Working from home too many days in a row.
  Avoiding people with whom I'm frustrated.

- What antidepressant behaviors do I need to maintain or increase?
  The main thing is social engagement. I need to stay in touch with my friends, even if I am feeling low and only call a friend and chat for a few minutes. I don't need to talk about my depression but can ask how things are going for them. I can say if I'm having a hard time, but I don't need to divulge details.
  Keeping physically active and doing things that I enjoy is really important—walking the dog or working in the garden.
  I also need to keep my apartment clean.
  Attending church on occasion is also good for me.
  Going into the office to work is also better for me than working from home when I am feeling down or starting to slip into feeling down.
  Using problem solving to resolve conflict that comes up at work or talking it over with a friend.
  Breaking down tasks that feel overwhelming to me, taking one step.
  It helps when I stop and think before talking when I am anxious.

- What can I do to increase the chances that I will follow through on my antidepressant behaviors?
  Keep a daily schedule in which each morning I write down the key activities to help my mood that I will do that day.
  Sign up for a class at the gym to help me stay on track with my exercise plan.
  Tell my boss now that I will be going to work every weekday, even though it's okay for me to telecommute.
  Work for at least 5 hours a day so that the workload does not accumulate.
  Schedule weekly check-ins now with my boss so that I have a place to address conflicts if they come up.
  Make contact with at least one friend every week. Tell two friends that I am committing to do this, and ask them to check in with me.
  During the spring, summer, and fall months, I will go to the pea patch at least once on the weekend, when the weather permits.

FIGURE 9.1. Alicia's notebook and posttherapy plan.

to understand the antecedents and consequences of behavior, acting from the "outside-in" rather than according to mood, and countering avoidance and rumination with specific activation tasks.

Expanding Activation to New Life Contexts and Goals after Treatment Ends

Teaching clients to activate in the face of depression, to recognize and modify avoidance behaviors, and to maintain healthy routines are core ingredients of BA. One of the basic assumptions of BA is that clients will be protected from relapse by making changes that help them build antidepressant lives. Although much of this work happens over the course of therapy for most clients, important changes will continue to be a focus of effort after therapy ends.

When clients have experienced symptom relief and are increasing activities and modifying avoidance behaviors, they may then be ready to tackle larger problems in the context of their lives. For instance, early in therapy Alicia and her therapist recognized how avoiding many activities exacerbated her sense of guilt and isolation. As therapy progressed, Alicia learned that taking small steps toward important goals when she felt down was better than taking no steps at all. She developed a new habit of taking her dog for a short walk and chatting casually with other dog walkers in the neighborhood, and she began to call friends to simply check in. In these ways, Alicia worked on changing the problem of isolation and loneliness that characterized her interpersonal life. As therapy progressed, she also began to address the problems in her work context. Beth helped Alicia identify the types of jobs she would like to pursue, the salary ranges she could consider that would allow her to move to a neighborhood she could enjoy, and inexpensive options for training that would keep Alicia's skills current and increase her qualifications for interesting work. Although Alicia began this work during the later phases of therapy, it also was critical for Beth to help Alicia continue such efforts after therapy ended.

It is important for therapists to help clients evaluate what changes may be required across multiple life contexts in order to support positive mood and well-being over time. Interpersonal relationships, employment, recreational or educational domains, and financial and housing issues can be considered. The therapist can help the client begin to identify goals and steps to reach those goals in these life domains. In their final sessions, for example, Beth and Alicia identified important steps that would be required to find the job she most wanted and what would be required to support such steps after therapy had ended. They also began to explore what long-term changes Alicia wanted to implement in her interpersonal relationships. In what ways was she satisfied or dissatisfied with her social life? Alicia discussed her hope that she would someday find a romantic partner and perhaps get married and have children. Although this possibility appeared to loom far into the future for Alicia, she described feeling lonely at times when she would see families enjoying time together at the park or in restaurants. She expressed a sense of longing to have these intimate connections in her life at some later point. "I know I'm not there now," she explained to Beth, "but once I get this other stuff together—my work, where I live, all that we have been working on—I know I want to have a family in my life, too." Together they explored how Alicia could apply the new behaviors she had learned in responding to her friends, employer, and coworkers in the context of pursuing intimate relationships.

Identifying and Preparing for High-Risk Situations

In preparation for ending BA, it is critical to identify potential high-risk situations for clients that may increase their vulnerability to relapse in the future. Key questions to ask about such situations include: "When is this most likely to occur?" "What can you do, if anything, to prevent this from happening?" "If this does happen, what are possible consequences and what can you do to reduce the impact?" (Wilson, 1992, p. 147).

Returning to the case formulation can be of enormous assistance in the process of identifying high-risk situations. Life events that preceded previous depressive episodes may provide clues to future possible high-risk situations. Let's consider Alicia's experience. Three precipitants to Alicia's depression were being laid off from her job, taking a lower-level job that she found boring, and moving into a small apartment. These situations suggest that Alicia may be susceptible to situations that involve a loss of status, possible criticism from friends or relatives, or a reduction in her ability to obtain effort-based rewards (for example, if she were to be ill or injured and less able to work in the garden or take walks). She also was unhappy about her living situation because the apartment was small, in an undesirable neighborhood, and reminded her of a place she had lived in during college—it felt like a step backward. Additionally, then, situations that were strong reminders of events that had transpired earlier in her life—for example, tapping strong emotions about her early relationship with her mother—might also be high-risk for her. Alicia and Beth identified her vulnerability to these types of contexts and clarified the possible high-risk situations that might result in these types of losses and have a similar negative impact in the future.

A typical course of BA helps clients generate a great deal of information that can inform answers to questions about combating depression in the future. A review of activity monitoring charts reveals situations that are most closely connected with depressed or other negative moods. These data can be of great help when planning for future situations, and therapists can review some of the situations in the final sessions as a reminder to clients. For example, a client whose activity charts continued to show patterns of depressed mood at mid-day on weekends when he was at home alone watching television might list unstructured leisure time as a risky situation.

Therapists can also graph symptom fluctuations, with scores from such objective measures as the Beck Depression Inventory (BDI) and discuss the patterns observed over the course of treatment. Figure 9.2 depicts Alicia's BDI-II scores as graphed over 18 sessions of therapy. When Beth presented her with the graph, they had a brief discussion about the pattern of scores, specific times that her mood

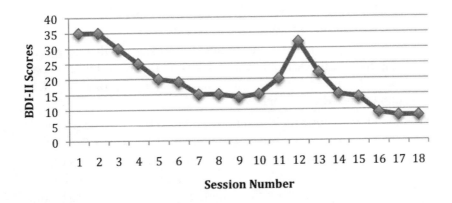

FIGURE 9.2. Alicia's BDI-II scores through session 18.

deteriorated during treatment, and what could be learned from this to anticipate future risk and helpful strategies.

BETH: Alicia, I've included on this graph the scores from the questionnaires you fill out at each of our sessions. I'm curious about any impressions you have as you look over this.

ALICIA: It looks a lot better now than when I first came in!

BETH: I agree! It's been a big change over time. Do you notice anything in particular that surprises you as you look at the patterns over the course of our work together?

ALICIA: Nothing that surprises me, but it does look like things got worse for a while.

BETH: I was struck by that, too. In fact, I looked back at my notes before we met today. During the period when your scores were highest, around our 12th session, you had reported that you were feeling like you were just "going through the motions" and you had avoided going to several events.

ALICIA: I remember that. Isn't that also when I missed a session?

BETH: Yes, it was when you had that stressful experience at work and then spent a day in bed.

ALICIA: That was really hard. I felt really badly during that time.

BETH: Yes, I'm thinking that one of the ways we can learn from this graph is to identify specific ways in which your mood may be vulnerable in the future and what you can do about it.

ALICIA: Well, I think that was when my boss was really harsh after I screwed up that project.

BETH: So, when you don't accomplish important goals and receive negative feedback from others is a time that you might be particularly vulnerable. Do you want to make a list of these? Why don't you write that one down?

ALICIA: That's a good idea. You know, it's also true that staying home and missing therapy wasn't the best idea then, either.

BETH: I was thinking that too. We've talked a lot about how withdrawing and avoiding can start that cycle of depression and keep it going over time. I am thinking that you are likely to feel worse if you stay in bed or avoid social commitments—like therapy then, but it could be plans with friends or coworkers too, right?

ALICIA: I guess that is probably the case. I remember that I felt more depressed after missing things.

BETH: So, this may be something to keep in mind in the future. When you are in one of those vulnerable times, like if you receive some critical feedback, continuing to engage instead of avoid is even more important. Let's talk about the specific activities you have learned to use to help you engage during those times. Do any come to mind?

ALICIA: Yes, probably coming up with small steps.

BETH: Absolutely! Even if you need to break down the activity to a bare minimum, rather than completely avoiding, you may prevent falling back into a depressed mood. Also, I think that what we've talked about in terms of attending to experience rather than ruminating might help during times when you feel like you are "going through the motions."

ALICIA: Yes, I agree. I'll write those ones down too.

Once several situations have been identified, the therapist and client work together to identify the ways in which one's behavioral antidepressant activities can be applied. For many clients, the active problem solving engaged in throughout therapy is likely to be a key ingredient. It is not necessary to ask clients to imagine every painful event possible, but if reasonable evidence exists that certain events will occur, coping strategies should be planned and ways in which the client might lessen the impact of the event can be planned. The plan should be as specific as possible, informed by what has worked during therapy, in order to support wellness and reduce risk over time.

Booster and Spaced Sessions

It often is helpful for clients to know that they can return for brief periods, or "booster sessions," in the future if they have slipped back into old patterns or are experiencing a period of depressive relapse. In particular, if clients begin to withdraw, lose interest in activities, and find they cannot pull out of it, this may be a time to reconnect briefly with the therapist. Several sessions can be scheduled to discuss current life stressors, review strategies that were helpful during the course of primary treatment, and make a game plan for coping.

It may also be useful to schedule maintenance sessions. While there are no data for BA, other cognitive and behavioral treatments have utilized maintenance sessions with good outcomes (Jarrett, Vittengl, & Clark, 2008). From this standpoint, it may be useful to increase the time frame between sessions as clients approach the end of a course of BA treatment. Spacing the sessions further apart allows the client to have more time to practice strategies that have been helpful and then return to troubleshoot with the therapist any difficulties experienced. Spacing final therapy sessions further apart also can allow for a broader array of situations to arise with which the client will need to cope. Spaced-out meetings with the therapist provide a refresher in planning strategies for continuing to engage and activate rather than avoiding and withdrawing from difficult situations.

Where Do We Go from Here?

Interest in BA and related behavioral treatments has been expanding rapidly in recent years. The clinical research on BA has provided added evidence that the early behavioral approach of Lewinsohn (1974) and colleagues (Lewinsohn et al., 1985) was on the right track in the effort to treat depression. Replication often being the hallmark of solid scientific research, it is noteworthy that the findings of Jacobson and colleagues' component analysis study (1996) that behavioral activation did as well as cognitive therapy were replicated in Dimidjian and colleagues' treatment for depression study (2006). Confidence in the efficacy of BA will be increased when those findings too are replicated in new settings, with new clinicians and patients, and by investigators who have not been involved in the development of the treatment.

Many important questions about BA remain to be addressed by future research. For example, because there are fewer techniques in BA than in other treatments for depression, it is possible that it is easier to learn and to disseminate to the clinical community. Empirical testing of this hypothesis awaits future research. We also know little about the ways in which BA achieves its effects. The mechanisms of change are difficult to identify. It is possible that clients in BA learn a new rule such as "When I feel depressed, I should get active rather than avoid." Perhaps clients in BA learn to take active control in their lives in ways that helps to produce immediate benefits and to protect themselves over time. The development of such other skills as setting goals and sequencing tasks may be critical. It also is possible that cognitive change is critical and that the best way to change a belief is through experience and behavior change (Bandura, 1977; Hollon, 2001). Undoubtedly, BA also has important effects on neural and other biological indices, which future research should be encouraged to explore.

Many new applications of BA also remain to be developed. Researchers currently are conducting small clinical trials using BA to address such problems as PTSD (Jakupcak et al., 2006; Wagner, Zatzick, Ghesquiere, & Jurkovich, 2007), and the use of BA as a transdiagnostic intervention may be substantiated in the future. Researchers also are exploring the application of BA within a multicultural framework. Currently BA has been adapted for work with Latino Americans (Santiago-Rivera et al., 2008), and the workbook by Addis and Martell (2004) has been translated into Swedish, Danish, and Dutch. Although the basic principles and strategies of BA may be useful across cultures, it is critical to examine the need for cultural specificity in the ways that therapists engage with clients; the concepts used and the emphasis on individualist versus collectivist understandings may vary in that context. Researchers are also conducting ongoing trials of BA across the lifespan, modifying the treatment protocols to be used with adolescents and elders.

Finally, there is increasing interest in applying BA in a group format. Such group delivery methods offer cost and efficiency advantages and are likely to be appealing in community mental health and other public health settings. One small study has demonstrated that BA can be conducted in this way (Houghton, Curran, & Saxon, 2008). The treatment mainly consisted of an adaptation of a BA self-help workbook (Addis & Martell, 2004) with the addition of a session focused on identifying values. The Addis and Martell workbook (2004) has served as the main organizing vehicle for most of the group sessions in these adapted designs. Future studies will likely explore a variety of group applications of the basic BA model.

These are exciting times for clinical researchers, as questions of both practical and theoretical importance demand investigation. Clinical practitioners can rest assured, however, that BA has a long history since the early 1970s, and the value of the activation has been underscored in numerous treatments over time. The principles and strategies that we have presented are likely to be of value for therapists who want to implement BA in its standard form with depressed clients. For therapists who utilize other models of treatment, it is likely that the elements of BA that we have discussed also will have some relevance and applicability. For example, behavioral activation is obviously a core part of cognitive therapy, and cognitive therapists can emphasize behavioral activation and feel confident that they are providing sound CBT. Acceptance and commitment therapists likely will find elements of value in their efforts to promote committed action with their clients. Dialectical behavior therapists will find much similarity between BA and basic strategies in DBT such as behavioral assessment, opposite action, and problem solving.

Often, upon attending a workshop on BA, therapists recognize many behaviors that are consistent with their current practices. Perhaps readers have recognized many of the clinical strategies that they use day in and day out as they have read this book. BA as a stand-alone approach may be the treatment of choice for many depressed clients, and for others the principles and strategies we have discussed will serve as a strong reminder to emphasize the behavioral aspects of treatment across a variety of contemporary therapies.

Putting It All Together

In this book we have covered the core principles and strategies of BA. If we were asked "What is the one thing that you hope clinicians will remember about BA?" our answer would be simple: activate. As an easy way for therapists to keep track of the core principles and strategies that support their efforts to activate clients skillfully, we offer a final acronym, ACTIVATE. In Appendix 4 we provide a quick reference for therapists. The letters represent the following processes that are essential to BA. BA therapists will do these things throughout treatment, namely: assess the factors contributing to the client's depression (A); counter avoidance with structured activation and effective problem solving (C); take time to get specific (T); include monitoring (I); validate (V); assign activities (A); troubleshoot (T); and encourage (E). These strategies do not need to be carried out in the order in which they are listed here. The practice of BA is not fixed and rigid, and therapists will make use of the interventions informed by the 10 core principles throughout treatment. This fluidity is illustrated by the fact that the core principles of BA enumerated in Table 2.1, page 23, do not follow in lockstep order with the interventions listed in the ACTIVATE acronym but rather are woven throughout. Let us consider each of the interventions in turn.

A: Assess

The importance of assessment throughout BA cannot be overstated. This element of BA has been emphasized throughout this book and in other publications about BA (e.g., Martell et al., 2001). Assessment is a primary focus of early sessions and throughout treatment. Assessment addresses the frequency and range of client activities as well as the function. Understanding the life circumstances that have contributed to a client's depression and also how the client has tried to cope with the depression provides initial insight into possible treatment targets (Principles 2 and 3). Knowing which behaviors to target as promising candidates for activation is accomplished through behavioral assessment of antecedents and consequences.

C: Counter Avoidance with Structured Activation and Effective Problem Solving

Depression often results from understandable reactions to negative life events that change reinforcement contingencies, reducing contact with reinforcers or increasing life problems. Avoidance and withdrawal are often sensible responses in the short term. Emotions have a strong momentum of their own, and negative moods both pull a person down and trigger attempts to avoid the feelings or life situations that feel overwhelming. The problem is that such avoidance and withdrawal behaviors often makes things worse in the long run, maintaining or exacerbating negative mood over time. Here we go back to Principle 1—one can change how one feels by changing what one does. Principle 4 is also key—structure and schedule activities that follow a plan, not a mood. BA works to help clients counter avoidance with structured activation and effective problem solving. Clients learn to identify their avoidance patterns and to have at the ready alternative coping strategies to support approach and engagement.

T: Take Time to Get Specific

The importance of behavioral specificity cannot be overstated. BA therapists help clients identify specific behaviors to be increased or decreased. Behaviors to increase are those that are likely to bring the client into contact with positive reinforcers in the environment, and those to decrease are ones that make the client's life more difficult in the long run.

I: Include Monitoring

Activity monitoring is a mainstay of BA. The activity chart is the primary tool used to support client monitoring of activities, context, mood or emotion, and intensity. Monitoring helps to make clear the context in which one's behavior is more or less likely to occur and the consequences of one's behavior, the awareness of which is a critical element of BA. Identifying these patterns is a central focus of therapy. Monitoring helps to inform action plans; without activity monitoring, it is difficult (if not impossible!) to identify effective targets for activation. Monitoring also informs the therapist and client whether action plans were effective and provides the information needed to tweak plans to be maximally helpful. Finally, the act of monitoring itself may help to promote change in behavior. Throughout treatment, we use monitoring as a core ingredient.

V: Validate

Being depressed often feels like being stuck in a very dark place with few means and little hope for escape. BA provides a way for many people suffering from depression to find their way back out of the dark to reengage and build a life they desire. During this process, it is critical for the BA therapist to be validating of the client, demonstrating an understanding of the client's experience and the challenges of change. Validation is the process of communicating that it makes perfect sense that the client sitting across the room feels and acts as he or she does in the moment *and* that efforts to change are critical if one is to feel better. Thus, the BA therapist coaches clients to experiment with different ways of activating and engaging that increase rewards and decrease aversive consequences in their lives—in a context of acceptance, warmth, collaboration, and encouragement.

A: Assign Activities

Activity scheduling and structuring are the primary ingredients of BA. The importance of assigning activities is reflected in many of the key principles of BA. As Principle 4 suggests, scheduling activities allows clients to have a clear plan to follow rather than falling into mood-dependent behaviors. Activity scheduling increases client engagement with the world, allowing greater contact with potential environmental positive reinforcement and opportunities to exert control over stressors. As Principle 5 implies, activities need to be assigned in steps and graded to increase the likelihood of success for the client. Principle 6 emphasizes that focusing in on these activities that have the greatest potential to produce change consists in finding those that are naturally reinforced in the client's environment and that have a high reward value. Finally, to remind the therapist of the central importance of activation, Principle 9 simply declares: don't just talk, do!

T: Troubleshoot

Most depressed clients experience challenges as they work to implement activation plans. Barriers arise and frustration can ensue. In order to keep therapy on track, Principle 10 reminds therapists to "Troubleshoot possible and actual barriers to activation." Troubleshooting is necessary to address the types of problems that commonly occur when developing and implementing activation plans with depressed clients. Therapists use troubleshooting to improve and tailor activation plans, and they teach clients how to troubleshoot on their own. Principle 8's advice to "Emphasize a problem-solving empirical approach, and recognize that all results are useful" is also instructive and relevant here, as the overall approach in BA is a problem-solving empirical one. Troubleshooting helps to make the best use of any client efforts aimed at activation and keeps therapy moving in the direction of the client's goals.

E: Encourage

The point at which most depressed clients seek professional help is the point at which they feel discouraged and demoralized. One of the ways that therapists maximize treatment success is by expressing consistently a sense of hope, optimism, and commitment to change. As Principle 7 states boldly, BA therapists are to function as coaches for clients, highlighting any signs of progress on the part of the client and encouraging any indicators or indications that the client is activating, engaging, and problem solving, particularly when he or she is feeling discouraged.

Summary

BA makes sense. The history of using these straightforward strategies with depressed clients has spanned nearly four decades since Lewinsohn (Lewinsohn & Graf, 1973) first wrote about "pleasant events" and depression. BA will undoubtedly continue to evolve, and future research will test its limits with new populations and problems. As therapists today, we can trust and confidently assert that BA is a proven and powerful method for helping people overcome the downward spiral of depression. It is rooted in behavioral principles that have withstood the test of time.

We have provided 10 "guiding principles" of BA—which we consider *core* ones—because we hope that therapists will be true to the empirically supported approach championed here and to the flexible and idiographic way in which it has been applied. BA therapists can respond to the individual situation of each client and remain activation-focused, guided by the core principles and strategies we have emphasized. Therapists—acting as coaches—and clients—doing the important work to activate—both benefit from following the principles. BA treatment must be done in a collaborative manner, therapists making suggestions and helping clients recognize when avoidance, reinforcement of depressed behavior, or disengagement from the environment inhibits antidepressant behavior.

At its heart, BA is pragmatic. Therapists may recognize their usual practices in the pages of this book. That is the elegance of the approach. We believe that BA is an easy treatment to learn because it is consistent with the practices of many clinicians working with depressed clients, it is straightforward, and the goal of helping clients to engage with their environments is a constant throughout treatment. Keeping one goal in mind during the process of collaboratively figuring out possible maintaining factors for clients' depression and barriers to change allows the therapy to keep from going astray in multiple directions. The focus is on the environment and on behavioral change. Therapists can easily recognize that helping depressed clients to increase activity is an important initial step in treatment, and the mounting evidence in support of BA suggests that it is a sufficient step. As active coaches in their behalf, therapists following the principles presented here will maintain a therapeutic stance that builds a strong connection to clients through the challenging and rewarding endeavor of creating a context for lasting positive change in their lives.

APPENDIX 1

Charts and Worksheets
for Depressed Clients

The following are charts that therapists may find helpful in their work with depressed clients.

Appendix 1a is a case conceptualization chart that the therapist and client can use to develop the individualized BA conceptualization. Appendix 1b is an activity and emotion monitoring chart. The client is asked to write down the emotion experienced as well as its intensity. Appendix 1c is an activity and mood monitoring chart. This chart is to be used to monitor the intensity of a client's depression. Appendix 1d is a chart for monitoring or scheduling activities and rating the amount of mastery or pleasure the activity provides. Appendices 1e and 1f provide formats for planning or scheduling activities. A TRAP-TRAC sheet is provided in Appendix 1g for clients to record when they experience avoidance and determine alternative coping to counter avoidant behavior. Appendix 1h is an ACTION sheet for clients to use to help them assess the function of their behavior and choose an action plan.

APPENDIX 1a

The Behavioral Activation Depression Model

Use this form to keep track of how changes in life (1) impact how rewarding or stressful life has become (2). How do you react to this (3)? What do you do to cope (4)? What impact do these behaviors have on the rewards and stressors in your life (5)?

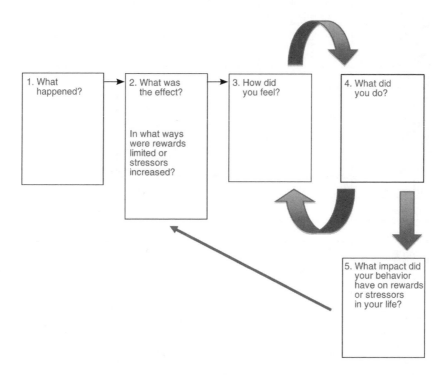

APPENDIX 1b

Behavioral Activation Activity Chart— Monitoring Activity and Emotion

Instructions: Record your activity for each hour of the day (what were you doing, with whom, where, etc.). Record an emotion associated with each activity (e.g., sad, happy, scared, angry, ashamed, disgusted, surprised). Rate your intensity of feeling between 1 and 10, with "1" = "not at all intense" and "10" = "very intense."

	Sun.	Mon.	Tues.	Wed.	Thurs.	Fri.	Sat.
5:00 A.M.–7:00 A.M.							
7:00 A.M.							
8:00 A.M.							
9:00 A.M.							
10:00 A.M.							
11:00 A.M.							
12:00 A.M.							
1:00 A.M.							
2:00 P.M.							
3:00 P.M.							
4:00 P.M.							
5:00 P.M.							
6:00 P.M.							
7:00 P.M.							
8:00 P.M.							
9:00 P.M.							
10:00 P.M.							
11:00 P.M.–5:00 A.M.							

APPENDIX 1c

Behavioral Activation Activity Chart— Monitoring Activity and Mood

Instructions: Record your activity for each hour of the day (what were you doing, with whom, where, etc.). Rate the intensity of your mood (i.e., how depressed you feel) between 1 and 10, with "1" = "not at all intense" and "10" = "very intense."

	Sun.	Mon.	Tues.	Wed.	Thurs.	Fri.	Sat.
5:00 A.M.–7:00 A.M.							
7:00 A.M.							
8:00 A.M.							
9:00 A.M.							
10:00 A.M.							
11:00 A.M.							
12:00 A.M.							
1:00 A.M.							
2:00 P.M.							
3:00 P.M.							
4:00 P.M.							
5:00 P.M.							
6:00 P.M.							
7:00 P.M.							
8:00 P.M.							
9:00 P.M.							
10:00 P.M.							
11:00 P.M.–5:00 A.M.							

Behavioral Activation Activity Chart—
Monitoring Activity/Pleasure/Mastery

Instructions: Record your activity for each hour of the day (what were you doing, with whom, where, etc.). Record a rating for the pleasure ("P") and the mastery ("M") that you experienced as you were doing each activity. Pleasure and mastery are each rated between 1 and 10, with "0" = "low" and "10" = "high."

	Sun.	Mon.	Tues.	Wed.	Thurs.	Fri.	Sat.
5:00 A.M.–7:00 A.M.							
7:00 A.M.							
8:00 A.M.							
9:00 A.M.							
10:00 A.M.							
11:00 A.M.							
12:00 A.M.							
1:00 A.M.							
2:00 P.M.							
3:00 P.M.							
4:00 P.M.							
5:00 P.M.							
6:00 P.M.							
7:00 P.M.							
8:00 P.M.							
9:00 P.M.							
10:00 P.M.							
11:00 P.M.–5:00 A.M.							

APPENDIX 1e

Behavioral Activation Activity Chart— Planned Activities

Instructions: Record the specific activities that you and your therapist agreed you would do this week in each of the rows (Activities 1–4). You do not need to use all of these rows, or you can add more rows, depending on the specific activities you plan for the week. For each day, place a check mark to indicate if you engaged in the assigned activity. Record a mood rating for each day in the last row; mood is rated between 1 and 10, with "1" = "not at all depressed" and "10" = "most severely depressed."

	Mon.	Tues.	Wed.	Thurs.	Fri.	Sat.	Sun.
Activity 1:							
Activity 2:							
Activity 3:							
Activity 4:							
Daily mood rating							

APPENDIX 1f

Behavioral Activation Activity Chart—
Scheduled Activities for _____

(list day of week/date)

Instructions: Schedule the specific activities that you and your therapist agreed you would do in the "Activity" column. Place a check mark in the "Completed" column to indicate if you completed the scheduled activity. Record a mood rating in the last column; mood is rated between 1 and 10, with "1" = "not at all depressed" and "10" = "most severely depressed.")

	Activity	Completed	Mood rating
5:00 A.M.– 7:00 A.M.			
7:00 A.M.			
8:00 A.M.			
9:00 A.M.			
10:00 A.M.			
11:00 A.M.			
12:00 A.M.			
1:00 A.M.			
2:00 P.M.			
3:00 P.M.			
4:00 P.M.			
5:00 P.M.			
6:00 P.M.			
7:00 P.M.			
8:00 P.M.			
9:00 P.M.			
10:00 P.M.			
11:00 P.M.– 5:00 A.M.			

APPENDIX 1g

TRAP-TRAC Sheet

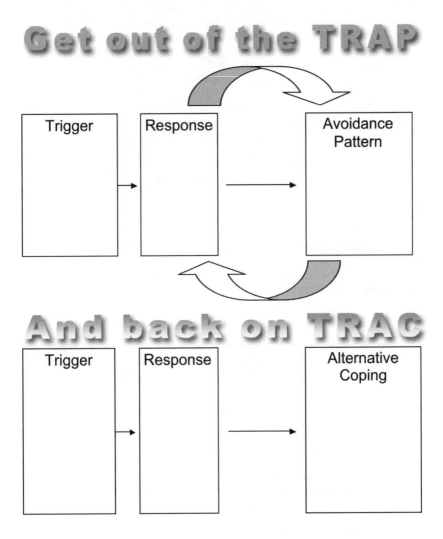

The ACTION Acronym—Client Version

Assess the function of a behavior. How is this behavior serving you? What are the consequences? Does the behavior act as a depressant? Is it inconsistent with long-term goals? Does the behavior act as an antidepressant? Is it consistent with long-term goals?

_____

_____

_____

_____

Choose an action. What action did you choose?

_____

_____

Try the behavior chosen. Record the specifics of your plan for putting the new behavior(s) into action.

_____

_____

Integrate new behavior(s) into a routine. If you are trying something new or engaging in behavior that is opposite to your mood, it is important to try more than once before concluding whether this is helpful or not. Integrate this into a normal routine. How will you do this?

_____

_____

Observe the results. What is the outcome? Do you feel better or worse after the action you chose to take? Has the action moved you closer to any of your goals? Have you integrated a new routine into your schedule? What changes do you notice?

_____

_____

_____

_____

Never give up. Repeat the steps above. Developing a new habit of activating and engaging requires repeated efforts. Over time, these antidepressant behaviors will become automatic, even when you are feeling down.

_____

Adapted from Martell, Addis, and Jacobson (2001, pp. 102–105) in *Behavioral Activation for Depression: A Clinician's Guide* by Christopher R. Martell, Sona Dimidjian, and Ruth Herman-Dunn (The Guilford Press, 2010). Permission to photocopy this form is granted to purchasers of this book for personal use only (see copyright page for details). Purchasers may download a larger version of this table from the book's page on The Guilford Press website.

APPENDIX 2

Notebook and Weekly Therapy Plan

These sheets can be used during your therapy or as a means of self-help to continue when therapy is completed.

Session Date: _____

- What problems were discussed today in therapy?

- What have I learned about the connections between how I feel and the activities in which I'm engaged?

- What behaviors do I need to increase that are antidepressant for me?

- When will I engage in these behaviors?

- Have I broken these behaviors into steps that I'm likely to complete?
  - If so, what are the steps?

- What activities have a good chance of being powerful enough for me to lose myself in?

- Are there any activities that I'm trying to escape or avoid?

- Are there any behaviors I need to decrease because they act as a depressant for me and are inconsistent with my long-term goals?

- To what stimuli or activities can I attend so as not to be stuck in my head?

- Where am I likely to have a particularly hard time?

- What can I do to make it likely that I'll be able to cope?

APPENDIX 3

Notebook and Posttherapy Plan

Answer the following questions to help you with a plan for managing moods and feelings and remaining engaged following the completion of therapy.

• What contexts increase my vulnerability to depression?

• What behaviors contribute to keeping the depression cycle going?

• What antidepressant behaviors do I need to maintain or increase?

• What can I do to increase the chances that I will follow through on my antidepressant behaviors?

201

APPENDIX 4

ACTIVATE Reference Sheet for Therapists

Assess

Assess the life situations that may be associated with the client's depression as well as the secondary problem behaviors that have developed as the client has tried to cope with depression.

Assess ongoing behaviors, using activity and mood monitoring charts as well as behavioral analysis.

Follow these principles:
- Changes in life can lead to depression, and efforts to cope that provide relief in the short term may keep you stuck over time (Principle 2).
- The clues to figuring out what is going to be antidepressant lie in noticing what precedes and what follows important behaviors (Principle 3).

Counter Avoidance with Structured Activation and Effective Problem Solving

A common function of depressed clients' behavior is escape and avoidance.

Using a problem-solving strategy and teaching clients to problem-solve can provide effective ways to counter avoidance.

Follow these principles:
- You can change how you feel by changing what you do (Principle 1).
- Structure and schedule activities in order to follow a plan, not a mood (Principle 4).

Take Time to Get Specific

Define and describe behavior in specific detail.

Define problems behaviorally.

Be concrete.

Include Monitoring

Use activity and mood monitoring charts to track client behaviors and progress.

Teach clients to monitor their own behavior by using written forms or other methods preferable to them.

Validate

The BA therapist validates the client's experience, always communicating an understanding of his or her actions and feelings.

The BA therapist is constantly responsive to the client.

The BA therapist is nonjudgmental and matter-of-fact.

Assign Activities
    Assign activities by using activity charts.
    Set goals with the client.
    Assign activities in steps.

Follow these principles:
- Structure and schedule activities in order to follow a plan, not a mood (Principle 4).
- Change is easier when you start small (Principle 5).
- Emphasize activities that are naturally reinforcing (Principle 6).
- Don't just talk, do! (Principle 9).

Troubleshoot
    There will be barriers to change. The therapist uses troubleshooting in the session to help overcome barriers, and he or she teaches the client to troubleshoot.

Follow these principles:
- Emphasize a problem-solving empirical approach, and recognize that all results are useful (Principle 8).
- Troubleshoot possible and actual barriers to activation (Principle 10).

Encourage
    The BA therapist encourages clients to work from the outside-in.
    The BA therapist remains optimistic.

Follow this principle:
- Act as a coach (Principle 7).

References

Addis, M. E., & Martell, C. R. (2004). *Overcoming depression one step at a time: The new behavioral activation treatment to getting your life back.* Oakland, CA: New Harbinger.

American Psychiatric Association Workgroup on Major Depressive Disorder. (2000). *Practice guideline for the treatment of patients with major depressive disorder.* Washington DC: American Psychiatric Association. Available at *www.psych.org/psych_pract/treatg/pg/Depression2e.book.cfm.*

Antony, M. M., Orsillo, S. M., & Roemer, L. (2001). *Practitioner's guide to empirically based measures of anxiety.* New York: Kluwer Academic/Plenum.

Bandura, A. (1977). *Social learning theory.* Englewood Cliffs, NJ: Prentice-Hall.

Bandura, A., & Schunk, D. H. (1981). Cultivating competence, self-efficacy, and intrinsic interest through proximal self-motivation. *Journal of Personality and Social Psychology, 41*(3), 586–598.

Barlow, D. H., Allen, L. B., & Choate, M. L (2004). Toward a unified treatment of Emotional disorders. *Behavior Therapy, 35,* 205–230.

Beck, A. T., Epstein, N., Brown, G., & Steer, R. A. (1988). An inventory for measuring clinical anxiety. *Journal of Consulting and Clinical Psychology, 56,* 893–897.

Beck, A. T., Rush, A. J., Shaw, B. F., & Emery, G. (1979). *Cognitive therapy of depression.* New York: Guilford Press.

Beck, A. T., & Steer, R. A. (1987). *Beck Depression Inventory: Manual.* San Antonio, TX: Psychological Corporation.

Beck, J. S. (1995). *Cognitive therapy: Basics and beyond.* New York: Guilford Press.

Biglan, A., & Dow, M. G. (1981). Toward a second-generation model: A

Problem-specific approach. In L. P. Rehm (Ed.), *Behavior therapy for depression: Present status and future directions* (pp. 97–121). New York: Academic Press.

Blustein, D. L. (2008). The role of work in psychological health and well-being. *American Psychologist, 63,* 228–240.

Bongar, B. (2002). *The suicidal patient: Clinical and legal standards of care* (2nd ed.). Washington, DC: American Psychological Association.

Borkovec, T. D., Alcaine, O. M., & Behar, E. (2004). Avoidance theory of worry and generalized anxiety disorder. In R. G. Heimberg, C. L. Turk, & D. S. Mennin (Eds.), *Generalized anxiety disorder: Advances in research and practice* (pp. 77–108). New York: Guilford Press.

Brown, J. D., & Siegel, J. M. (1988). Attributions for negative life events and depression: The role of perceived control. *Journal of Personality and Social Psychology, 54*(2), 316–322.

Brown, W. J., Ford, J. H., Burton, N. W., Marshall, A. L., & Dobson, A. J. (2005). Prospective study of physical activity and depressive symptoms in middle-aged women. *American Journal of Preventive Medicine, 29*(14), 265–272.

Caldwell, L. L. (2005). Leisure and health: Why is leisure therapeutic? *British Journal of Guidance and Counselling, 33*(1), 7–26.

Chomsky, N. (1959). A review of B. F. Skinner's *Verbal Behavior. Language, 35,* 26–58.

Chung, J. C. C. (2004). Activity participation and well-being of people with dementia in long-term-care settings. *OTJR: Occupation, Participation, and Health, 24*(1), 22–31.

Dahl, J. C., Plumb, J. C., Stewart, I., & Lundgren, T. (2009). *The art and science of valuing in psychotherapy: Helping clients discover, explore, and commit to valued action using acceptance and commitment therapy.* Oakland, CA: New Harbinger.

DeRubeis, R. J., Hollon, S. D., Amsterdam, J. D., Shelton, R. C., Young, P. R., Salomon, R. M., et al. (2005). Cognitive therapy vs. medications in the treatment of moderate to severe depression. *Archives of General Psychiatry, 62,* 409–416.

DeRubeis, R. J., Siegle, G. J., & Hollon ,S. D. (2008). Cognitive therapy versus medication for depression: Treatment outcomes and neural mechanisms. *Nature Reviews Neuroscience, 9,* Article 10. Retrieved March 13, 2009, from *www.nature.com/nrn/journal/v9/n10/index.html.*

Dimidjian, S. (2000, June 2). Skepticism, compassion, and the treatment of depression. *Prevention and Treatment, 3,* Article 26. Retrieved March 10, 2009, from *journals.apa.org/pt/prevention/volume3/pre0030026c.html.*

Dimidjian, S., Hollon, S. D., Dobson, K. S., Schmaling, K. B., Kohlenberg, R. J., Addis, M. E., et al. (2006). Randomized trial of behavioral activation, cognitive therapy, and antidepressant medication in the acute treatment of adults with major depression. *Journal of Consulting and Clinical Psychology, 74*(4), 658–670.

Dimidjian, S., Martell, C. R., Addis, M. E., & Herman-Dunn, R. (2008). Behavioral activation for depression. In D. H. Barlow (Ed.), *Clinical handbook of psychological disorders* (4th ed.): *A step-by-step treatment manual* (pp. 328–364). New York: Guilford Press.

Dishman, R. K., Berthoud, H.-R., Booth, F. W., Cotman, C. W., Edgerton, V. R., Fleshner, M. R., et al. (2006). Neurobiology of exercise. *Obesity, 14,* 345–356.

Dobson, K. S., Hollon, S. D., Dimidjian, S., Schmaling, K. B., Kohlenberg, R. J., Gallop, R. J., et al. (2008). Randomized trial of behavioral activation, cognitive therapy, and antidepressant medication in the prevention of relapse and recurrence in major depression. *Journal of Consulting and Clinical Psychology, 76*(3), 468–477.

Dunn, A. L., Trivedi, M. H., Kampert, J. B., Clark, C. G., & Chambliss, H. O. (2005). Exercise treatment for depression: Efficacy and dose–response. *American Journal of Preventive Medicine, 28*(1), 1–8.

D'Zurilla, T. J., & Goldfried, M. R. (1971). Problem solving and behavior modification. *Journal of Abnormal Psychology, 78,* 107–128.

D'Zurilla, T. J., & Nezu, A. M. (1982). Social problem solving in adults. In P. C. Kendall (Ed.), *Advances in cognitive-behavioral research and therapy* (Vol. 1, pp. 201–274). New York: Academic Press.

D'Zurilla, T. J., & Nezu, A. M. (1999). *Problem-solving therapy: A social competence approach to clinical intervention* (2nd ed.). New York: Springer.

Elkin, I., Shea, T., Watkins, J. T., Imber, S. C., Sotsky, S. M., Collins, J. F., et al. (1989). NIMH Treatment of Depression Collaborative Research Program. *Archives of General Psychiatry, 46,* 971–982.

Ferster, C. B. (1973). A functional analysis of depression. *American Psychologist, 28,* 857–870.

Ferster, C. B. (1974). Behavioral approaches to depression. In R. J. Friedman & M. M. Katz (Eds.), *The psychology of depression: Contemporary theory and research* (pp. 29–45). Washington, DC: New Hemisphere.

Fossati, P., Ergis, A.-M., & Allilaire, J. F. (2001). Problem-solving abilities in unipolar depressed patients: Comparison of performance on the modified version of the Wisconsin and the California sorting tests. *Psychiatry Research, 104,* 145–156.

Fuchs, C. Z., & Rehm, L. P. (1977). A self-control behavior therapy program for depression. *Journal of Consulting and Clinical Psychology, 45,* 206–215.

Furmark, T., Tillfors, M., Marteinsdottier, I., Fischer, H., Pissiota, A., Långström, B., et al. (2002). Common changes in cerebral blood flow in patients with social phobia treated with citalopram or cognitive-behavioral therapy. *Archives of General Psychiatry, 59,* 425–433.

Goldapple, K., Segal, Z., Garson, C., Lau, M., Bieling, P., Kennedy, H., et al. (2004). Modulation of cortical-limbic pathways in major depression. *Archives of General Psychiatry, 61,* 34–41.

Gollwitzer, P. M. (1999). Implementation intentions: Strong effects of simple plans. *American Psychologist, 54,* 493–503.

Gollwitzer, P. M., & Brandstätter, V. (1997). Implementation intentions and effective goal pursuit. *Journal of Personality and Social Psychology, 73,* 186–199.

Gortner, E. T., Gollan, J. K., Dobson, K. S., & Jacobson, N. S. (1998). Cognitive-behavioral treatment for depression: Relapse prevention. *Journal of Consulting and Clinical Psychology, 66*(2), 377–384.

Gotlib, I. H., & Asarnow, R. F. (1979). Interpersonal and impersonal problem-solving skills in mildly and clinically depressed university students. *Journal of Consulting and Clinical Psychology, 47,* 86–95.

Gray, J. (1982). *The neuropsychology of anxiety: An enquiry into the functions of the septo-hippocampal system.* Oxford, UK: Oxford University Press.

Hayes, S. C., Barnes-Holmes, D., & Roche, B. (2001). *Relational frame theory: A post-Skinnerian account of human language and cognition.* New York: Kluwer Academic/Plenum.

Hayes, S. C., & Brownstein, A. J. (1986). Mentalism, behavior–behavior relations, and a behavior-analytic view of the purposes of science. *The Behavior Analyst, 9,* 175–190.

Hayes, S. C., Luoma, J. B., Bond, F. W., Masuda, A., & Lillis, J. (2006). Acceptance and commitment therapy: Model, process and outcomes. *Behaviour Research and Therapy, 44,* 1–25.

Hayes, S. C., Strosahl, K. D., & Wilson, K. G. (1999). *Acceptance and commitment therapy: An experiential approach to behavior change.* New York: Guilford Press.

Hollon, S. D. (2001). Behavioral activation treatment for depression: A commentary. *Clinical Psychology: Science and Practice, 8*(3), 271–274.

Hollon, S. D., Jarrett, R. B., Nierenberg, A. A., Thase, M. E., Trivedi, M., & Rush, A. J. (2005). Psychotherapy and medication in the treatment of adult and geriatric depression: Which monotherapy or combined treatment? *Journal of Clinical Psychiatry, 66,* 455–468.

Hollon, S. D., Stewart, M. O., & Strunk, D. (2006). Enduring effects of cognitive behavior therapy in the treatment of depression and anxiety. *Annual Review of Psychiatry, 57,* 285–315.

Hollon, S. D., Thase, M. E., & Markowitz, J. C. (2002). Treatment and prevention of depression. *Psychological Science in the Public Interest, 3,* 39–77.

Hopko, D. R., Bell, J. L., Armento, M. E. A., Hunt, M. K., & Lejuez, C. W. (2005). Behavior therapy for depressed cancer patients in primary care. *Psychotherapy: Theory, Research, Practice, Training, 42,* 236–243.

Hopko, D. R., & Lejuez, C. W. (2007). *A cancer patient's guide to overcoming depression and anxiety: Getting through treatment and getting back to your life.* Oakland, CA: New Harbinger.

Hopko, D. R., Lejuez, C. W., & Hopko, S. D. (2004). Behavioral activation as an intervention for co-existent depressive and anxiety symptoms. *Clinical Case Studies, 3,* 37–48.

Hopko, D. R., Lejuez, C. W., LePage, J. P., Hopko, S. D., & McNeil, D. W. (2003). A brief behavioral activation treatment for depression: A randomized trial within an inpatient psychiatric hospital. *Behavior Modification, 27,* 458–469.

Hopko, D. R., Lejuez, C. W., Ruggiero, K. J., & Eifert, G. H. (2003). Contemporary behavioral activation treatments for depression: Procedures, principles, and progress. *Clinical Psychology Review, 23,* 699–717.

Houghton, S., Curran, J., & Saxon, D. (2008). An uncontrolled evaluation of group behavioural activation for depression. *Behavioural and Cognitive Psychotherapy, 36*(2), 235–239.

Jacobson, N. S., Dobson, K. S., Truax, P. A., Addis, M. E., Koerner, K., Gollan, J. K., et al. (1996). A component analysis of cognitive-behavioral therapy for depression. *Journal of Consulting and Clinical Psychology, 64*(2), 295–304.

Jacobson, N. S., & Gortner, E. T. (2000). Can depression be de-medicalized in the 21st century: Scientific revolutions, counter-revolutions and the magnetic field of normal science. *Behaviour Research and Therapy, 38,* 103–117.

Jacobson, N. S., & Margolin, G. (1979). *Marital therapy: Strategies based on social learning and behavior exchange principles.* New York: Brunner/Mazel.

Jacobson, N. S., Martell, C. R., & Dimidjian, S. (2001). Behavioral activation treatment for depression: Returning to contextual roots. *Clinical Psychology: Science and Practice, 8*(3), 255–270.

Jakupcak, M., Roberts, L. J., Martell, C. , Mulick, P., Michael, S., Reed, R., et al. (2006). A pilot study of behavioral activation for veterans with posttraumatic stress disorder. *Journal of Traumatic Stress, 19,* 387–391.

Jarrett, R. B., Vittengl, J. R., & Clark, L. A. (2008). Preventing recurrent depression. In M. A. Whisman (Ed.), *Adapting cognitive therapy for depression: Managing complexity and comorbidity* (pp. 132–156). New York: Guilford Press.

Jobes, D. A. (2006). *Managing suicidal risk: A collaborative approach.* New York: Guilford Press.

Kabat-Zinn, J. (1994). *Wherever you go, there you are: Mindfulness meditation in everyday life.* New York: Hyperion.

Kanfer, F. H. (1970). Self-regulation: Research issues and speculations. In C. Neuringer & J. L. Michael (Eds.), *Behavior modification in clinical psychology* (pp. 178–220). New York: Appleton-Century-Crofts. As cited in Rehm, L. P. (1977). A self-control model of depression. *Behavior Therapy, 8,* 787–804.

Lejuez, C. W., Hopko, D. R., LePage, J., Hopko, S. D., & McNeil, D. W. (2001). A brief behavioral activation treatment for depression. *Cognitive and Behavioral Practice, 8,* 164–175.

Lewinsohn, P. M. (1974). A behavioral approach to depression. In R. M. Friedman & M. M. Katz (Eds.), *The psychology of depression: Contemporary theory and research* (pp. 157–185). New York: Wiley.

Lewinsohn, P. M. (2001). Lewinsohn's model of depression. In W. E. Craighead & C. B. Nemeroff (Eds.), *The Corsini encyclopedia of psychology and behavioral science* (3rd ed., pp. 442–444). New York: Wiley.

Lewinsohn, P. M., Biglan, A., & Zeiss, A. S. (1976). Behavioral treatment of depression. In P. O. Davidson (Ed.), *The behavioral management of anxiety, depression and pain* (pp. 91–146). New York: Brunner/Mazel.

Lewinsohn, P. M., & Graf, M. (1973). Pleasant activities and depression. *Journal of Consulting and Clinical Psychology, 41,* 261–268.

Lewinsohn, P. M., Hoberman, H. M., Teri, L., & Hautzinger, M. (1985). An integrative theory of unipolar depression. In S. Reiss & R. R. Bootzin (Eds.), *Theoretical issues in behavioral therapy* (pp. 313–359). New York: Academic Press.

Lewinsohn, P. M., & Libet, J. (1972). Pleasant events, activity schedules and depressions. *Journal of Abnormal Psychology, 79,* 291–295.

Linehan, M. M. (1993). *Cognitive-behavioral treatment of borderline personality disorder.* New York: Guilford Press.

Linehan, M. M. (2006). Foreword. In A. M. Levinthal & C. R. Martell, *The myth of depression as disease: Limitations and alternatives to drugs* (pp. ix–xi). New York: Praeger.

Locke, E. A., & Latham, G. P. (1990). *A theory of goal setting and task performance.* Englewood Cliffs, NJ: Prentice-Hall.

Lucas, R. E., Clark, A. E., Georgellis, Y., & Diener, E. (2004). Unemployment alters the set-point for life satisfaction. *Psychological Science, 39,* 8–13.

Mace, F. C., & Kratochwill, T. R. (1985). Theories of reactivity in self-monitoring. *Behavior Modification, 9,* 323–343.

MacPhillamy, D. J., & Lewinsohn, P. M. (1982). The pleasant events schedule: Studies in reliability, validity, and scale intercorrelation. *Journal of Consulting and Clinical Psychology, 50,* 363–380.

Mallinckrodt, B., & Bennet, J. (1992). Social support and the impact of job loss in dislocated blue-collar workers. *Journal of Counseling Psychology, 39,* 482–489.

Marlatt, G. A., & Gordon, J. R. (1985). *Relapse prevention: Maintenance strategies in the treatment of addictive behaviors.* New York: Guilford Press.

Martell, C. R. (1988). Assessment of relevant stimuli affecting generalization in social skills training for retarded adults. *Dissertation Abstracts International,* 49(5-A), 1098.

Martell, C. R., Addis, M. E., & Jacobson, N. S. (2001). *Depression in context: Strategies for guided action.* New York: Norton.

Marzuk, P. M., Hartwell, N., Leon, A. C., & Portera, L. (2005). Executive functioning in depressed patients with suicidal ideation. *Acta Psychiatrica Scandinavica, 112,* 294–301.

Mather, A. S., Rodriguez, C., Guthrie, M. F., McHarg, A. M., Reid, I. C., & McMurdo, M. T. (2002). Effects of exercise on depressive symptoms in older adults with poor responsive depressive disorder: Randomized controlled trial. *British Journal of Psychiatry, 180,* 411–415.

Murphy, F. C., Rubinsztein, J. S., Michael, A., Rogers, R. D., Robbins, T. W., Paykel, E. S., et al. (2001). Decision-making cognition in mania and depression. *Psychological Medicine, 31,* 679–693.

Mynors-Wallis, L. M., Gath, D., Davies, I., Gray, A., & Barbour, F. (1997). A randomized controlled trial and cost analysis of problem-solving treatment given by community nurses for emotional disorders in primary care, *British Journal of Psychiatry, 170,* 113–119.

Nakatani, E., Nakgawa, A., Ohara, Y., Goto, S., Uozumi, N., Iwakiri, M., et al. (2003). Effects of behavior therapy on regional cerebral blood flow in obsessive-compulsive disorder. *Psychiatry Research: Neuroimaging, 124,* 113–120.

Nezu, A. M. (1987). A problem-solving formulation of depression: A literature review and proposal of a pluralistic model. *Clinical Psychology Review, 7,* 122–144.

Nezu, A. M. (2004). Problem solving and behavior therapy revisited. *Behavior Therapy, 35* 1–33.

Nezu, A. M., Ronan, G. F., Meadows, E. A., & McClure, K. S. (2000). *Practitioner's guide to empirically based measures of depression.* New York: Kluwer Academic/Plenum.

Nolen-Hoeksema, S. (2000). The role of rumination in depressive disorders and mixed anxiety/depressive symptoms. *Journal of Abnormal Psychology, 109,* 504–511.

Nolen-Hoeksema, S., Morrow, J., & Fredrickson, B. L. (1993). Response styles and the duration of episodes of depressed mood. *Journal of Abnormal Psychology, 102,* 20–28.

Nolen-Hoeksema, S., Parker, L., & Larson, J. (1994). Ruminative coping with depressed mood following a loss. *Journal of Personality and Social Psychology, 67,* 92–104.

Pavlov, I. (1927). *Conditioned reflexes* (G. V. Anrep, Trans.). London: Oxford University Press.

Premack, D. (1959). Toward empirical behavior laws: I. Positive reinforcement. *Psychological Review, 66,* 219–233.

Rehm, L. P. (1977). A self-control model of depression. *Behavior Therapy, 8,* 787–804.

Santiago-Rivera, A., Kanter, J., Benson, G., Derose, T., Illes, R., & Reyes, W. (2008). Behavioral activation as an alternative treatment approach for Latinos with depression. *Psychotherapy Research, Theory, Practice, Training, 45*(2), 173–185.

Schwartz, J. M., Stoessel, P. W., Baxter, L. R., Jr., Martin, K. M., & Phelps, M. E. (1996). Systematic changes in cerebral glucose metabolic rate after successful behavior modification treatment of obsessive–compulsive disorder. *Archives of General Psychiatry, 53,* 109–113.

Scogin, F., Jamison, C., & Gochneaur, K. (1989). Comparative efficacy of cognitive and behavioral bibliotherapy for mildly and moderately depressed older adults. *Journal of Consulting and Clinical Psychology, 57,* 403–407.

Segal, Z. V., Williams, J. M. G., & Teasdale, J. D. (2001). *Mindfulness-based cognitive therapy for depression: A new approach to preventing relapse.* New York: Guilford Press.

Seminowicz, D. A., Mayberg, B. S., McIntosh, A. R., Goldapple, K., Kennedy, S., Segal, Z., et al. (2004). Limbic-frontal circuitry in major depression: A path modeling meta-analysis. *NeuroImage, 22,* 409–418.

Shen, G. H. C., Alloy, L. B., Abramson, L. Y., & Sylvia, L. G. (2008). Social rhythm regularity and the onset of affective episodes in bipolar spectrum individuals. *Bipolar Disorders, 10,* 520–529.

Skinner, B. F. (1957). *Verbal behavior.* New York: Appleton-Century-Crofts.

Skinner, B. F. (1974). *About behaviorism.* New York: Knopf.

Stokes, T. F., & Baer, D. M. (1977). An implicit technology of generalization. *Journal of Applied Behavior Analysis, 10,* 349–367.

Sulzer-Azaroff, B., & Mayer, G. R. (1991). *Behavior analysis for lasting change.* New York: Holt, Rinehart and Winston.

Sutherland, A. (2008). *What Shamu taught me about life ,love ,and marriage: Lessons for people from animals and their trainers.* New York: Random House.

Treynor, W., Gonzalez, R., & Nolen-Hoeksema, S. (2003). Rumination reconsidered: A psychometric analysis. *Cognitive Therapy and Research, 27*(3), 247–259.

Valenstein, E. S. (1998). *Blaming the brain*. New York: Free Press.

Wagner, A. W., Zatzick, D. F., Ghesquiere, A., & Jurkovich, G. J. (2007). Behavioral activation as an early intervention for posttraumatic stress disorder and depression among physically injured trauma survivors. *Cognitive and Behavioral Practice, 14*, 341–349.

Warwar, S. H., Links, P. S., Greenberg, L., & Bergmans, Y. (2008). Emotion-focused principles for working with borderline personality disorder. *Journal of Psychiatric Practice, 14*, 94–104.

Watkins, E. R., Scott, J., Wingrove, J., Rimes, K. A., Bathurst, N., Steiner, H., et al. (2008). Rumination-focused cognitive behaviour therapy for residual depression: A case series. *Behaviour Research and Therapy, 45*, 2144–2154.

Watson, D. L., & Tharp, R. G. (2002). *Self-directed behavior: Self-modification for personal adjustment*. Belmont, CA: Wadsworth.

Watson, J., & Raynor, R. (1920). Conditioned emotional reactions. *Journal of Experimental Psychology, 3*, 1–14.

Williams, J. M. G., Teasdale, J. D., Segal, Z. V., & Kabat-Zinn, J. (2007). *The mindful way through depression: Freeing yourself from chronic unhappiness*. New York: Guilford Press.

Wilson, P. H. (1992). Depression. In P. H. Wilson (Ed.), *Principles and practice of relapse prevention* (pp. 128–156). New York: Guilford Press.

Wolpe, J. (1958). *Psychotherapy by reciprocal inhibition*. Stanford, CA: Stanford University Press.

Yoman, J. (2008). A primer on functional analysis. *Cognitive and Behavioral Practice, 15*, 325–340.

Zeiss, A. M., Lewinsohn, P. M., & Muñoz, R. F. (1979). Nonspecific improvement effects in depression using interpersonal skills training, pleasant activity schedules, or cognitive training. *Journal of Consulting and Clinical Psychology, 47*, 427–439.

Zettle, R. D., & Hayes, S. C. (1987). A component and process analysis of cognitive therapy. *Psychological Reports, 61*, 939–953.

Zettle, R. D., & Rains, J. C. (1989). Group cognitive and contextual therapies in treatment of depression. *Journal of Clinical Psychology, 45*(3), 436–445.

Index

Page numbers followed by an *f* or *t* indicate figures or tables.